Microtia
Sophie's Little Adventure

Dawn Calvert

Copyright © 2018 Dawn Calvert
All rights reserved.
No part of this book may be reproduced, stored in a retrieval system, or transmitted in any form, or by any means, electronic, mechanical, photocopying, recording or otherwise, without prior permission of the author.
ISBN-13: **978-1979722315**
ISBN-10: **1979722315**

DEDICATION

For Sophie

When I first saw you it only took a second to love you.
You are a very special little girl.
Thank you for enriching all our lives.

CONTENTS

1	Sophie Faith Ross	1
2	The Early Months	15
3	Microtia	39
4	Meeting Surgeons	55
5	Help!	79
6	Progress	89
7	Moving On	117
8	Looking Ahead	129
	Postscript	134
	Acknowledgements	136

Chapter 1

Sophie Faith Ross

Born Tues 7ᵗʰ December 2010 8lbs 10·5ozs

It was 8.45 pm that cold winter evening when my youngest daughter Fiona phoned me. She said, "Hi Granny, you have a beautiful baby grand-daughter!" I wasn't expecting this at all as she had gone to the hospital at 5 am that morning with her husband Colin because her waters had broken, and she had phoned me from the hospital around 4 pm saying that nothing much was happening, so it was a shock when she said the baby was born! My reply was, "That's brilliant, I can't believe it!" and I told her to hold on while I went into the living room to tell everyone.

My second eldest daughter Melanie and her French boyfriend Sam had arrived from New Zealand that afternoon and my eldest daughter Amanda was visiting us with her husband Mitch and children Noah and Megan. I shouted, "Fiona's had a little girl, Sophie Faith!" Everyone was elated and starting cheering! I put the phone to my ear again and said, "This is great Fiona, I can't believe you had her so quickly. What's she like?" Fiona said, "She's lovely with really dark hair, but mum, there's a wee problem." I felt my heart starting to pound and asked her what was wrong. She said, "Her wee ears haven't formed properly. There's no hole." My heart lurched as I struggled for something to say so I asked her what her ears were like. Fiona said they were folded over and when you pulled them back a bit there was no hole. I told her not to worry, that Sophie would be fine and there's bound to be something they can do. I told her not to panic until she found out more and that it was probably something simple like making new holes in her ears. Fiona then said she had to go as she had to get herself sorted out after the birth.

I really didn't know how I felt. One of my daughters came to me and I told her, then the others. No-one knew how to react. Everyone tried to be positive, we just hoped that it wasn't as bad as it sounded and that it could be sorted, but deep down we were all worried.

When Fiona fell pregnant it was unexpected, very exciting and a bit strange for me. This was my youngest, my baby girl going to have her own baby! How strange! It seemed not so long ago that she was born, the most beautiful baby in the hospital, (not only my thoughts, but those of the doctors and nurses also!). They all commented and marveled at how lovely she was and how perfect her features were! We have four lovely children, three girls and a boy, all born with no hitches. My husband Ronnie and I have always felt so fortunate to have such a lovely, complete family. Amanda our eldest child has two lovely children, Noah and Megan. I had two grandchildren and now another one on the way! Fiona's pregnancy was normal, she always looked and felt great. It never crossed my mind that there could be any problems. There was no reason to think otherwise.

Now here we are on 7th December 2010. Fiona's wee baby has been born and her ears have not developed properly. The reality that things can go wrong sank in. That evening the whole mood changed from elation to worry and concern for Fiona, Colin and their wee baby. We had only just met Sam, Melanie's French boyfriend, and that had been very exciting, so we had to try and be normal and continue to make him feel welcome. The rest of the evening was spent with mixed emotions, mixed vibes and mixed conversations. Poor Sam not only had to deal with the daunting task of meeting Melanie's family, trying to speak English and understand us at the same time, but he was also seeing a family coping with news that was both very exciting and upsetting at the same time.

My husband and I went to bed that night not really knowing what to say to each other. As I struggled to sleep my thoughts were with Fiona, Colin and their little baby girl. I so much wanted to be with them and tell them that everything would be alright. I just didn't want them to feel sad at a time that was supposed to be the happiest moment in their lives. When any of my children are sad and worried, I am also sad and worried and I would do anything to make them feel better. I couldn't even go to the hospital that night because they were so strict on visiting times, even with husbands and partners.

When we got up the next morning my husband said to me, "I went to bed thinking about wee Sophie and woke up thinking about her." I had the same thoughts. Visiting time was in the afternoon from 2-4 pm so Melanie and I decided to go then. When we went into the ward we saw a little baby girl who stood out because of her dark hair, dark eyes and sallow skin. She had these cute little ears which appeared to be folded over from the back and fixed to the side of her head. This was a baby who was beautiful in every sense and I fell in love with her straightaway. She was perfect and lovely just like her mum was when she was born. I gave Fiona and Colin a big hug but they both looked pale and drawn and were obviously putting on a brave face. I really felt for them, I knew they were worried, but then so was I but I had to be strong. I told them how beautiful she was and that things would work out. I had a close look at her ears and thought I saw a faint pinhole, a glimmer of hope that this wasn't as serious as it looked. I felt positive and said that hopefully the doctors will be able to pull back the ears and make a hole into the canal. Then Fiona asked, "Do you think she can hear?" This was the question we all wanted to ask but were afraid to. Is Sophie deaf? Will she ever be able to hear? I just had to say I didn't know. Fiona and Colin were holding it together but the pain was written all over their faces. They didn't want this for their baby, none of us wanted it. As parents we never want anything to be wrong with our children, but this time something was wrong and now we had to deal with it. I had to be strong for everyone no matter how I felt inside. This is what being a mother is all about, and I knew this would be how Fiona would feel about Sophie as she grew up. That afternoon we all nursed Sophie while Fiona told us about the birth. Colin told us a few stories about Fiona's antics while under the influence of 'gas and air' and this made us laugh. We took some photos too and managed to relax a bit. They said a paediatrician was coming to see Sophie later on and hopefully they would know more then. The midwife told them she had only ever seen this condition once before and had no idea what it was. Finally Melanie and I had to leave. I told Fiona we would get through this together. Sophie was truly a beautiful and special baby.

When we arrived back home I was slightly more upbeat and convinced that things were not as bad as they looked. I remember I had made Chilli con Carne for dinner that evening. There were just the four of us, Melanie, Sam, my husband and myself. I was getting ready to serve out the dinner when the phone rang. It

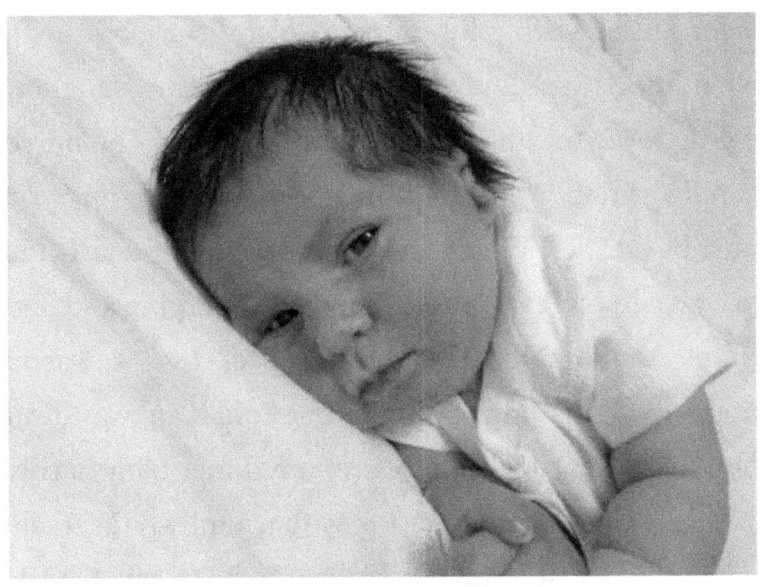

Figure 1: Sophie, 1 day old

was Fiona. She said that the paediatrician had come to see Sophie and said that as her outer ears hadn't formed properly it was highly unlikely that her inner ears would have formed. When he examined her he said she had no ear canal. I was devastated and asked Fiona what they were going to do. She said that Sophie was being referred to a consultant from the ENT department of the hospital the next day. Fiona was very upset and was crying. She said, "I was holding her and talking to her, but what's the point, she can't even hear me." I said that she must keep talking to her and interacting with her even if she can't hear, because she needs to see visible interaction so she can bond with her mum. I was doing my best to make my daughter feel better. I told her that Sophie would be ok and so would she and Colin. "Sophie needs you both and you must be strong." Who was I to give advice? I nearly fell apart when I put the phone down. I was crying and had to tell the others. They were upset too. I wasn't interested in serving up dinner but I did it anyway even though I didn't feel like eating anything. Sam hardly spoke, he was in this situation with a family he scarcely knew and he just didn't know what to do or say. I really felt sorry for him because we couldn't be our normal selves on his first visit to Belfast. I tried to hold it together through dinner but the tears were flowing while I was eating. Sam didn't finish his dinner and he told Melanie later that it was because he felt so sad for everyone. Then I had to phone Amanda and my mum and tell them that Sophie's problem was more serious than we thought and that she was probably deaf. Our only son Simon was in Australia and not due home for Christmas until 21st December so I had to text him the news. He was gutted and very sad and felt isolated because he was so far away from his family with no-one to talk to.

That Wednesday was one of the worst and saddest days of my life. It was even worse than the day we were told my husband had MS because we were more prepared for that and knew for a long time that he probably had it. The news about Sophie's ears was sudden and threw us all into turmoil and we couldn't believe it had happened. Don't get me wrong, we were so very thankful for this lovely baby and she was already loved so much by everyone, but we are all only human and deep down we were devastated about her ears, devastated for Fiona and Colin and devastated that it had happened. I think we wouldn't be normal and honest if we said we didn't feel like this. Looking back I wonder did we react normally, but I think we did. It is the fact of being in unknown territory and having this fear of handling it then and in the future, that throws your life into disarray.

Thursday 9th December was the day they had to see the ENT specialist. The appointment was supposed to be in the early afternoon so I thought that by the time I got to the hospital they would have seen him and had some news for me. When I arrived they were still waiting to be called down for the consultation so they asked me to go with them, which I was pleased about.

The specialist came across as a very nice man and took Sophie from Fiona to examine her ears. He then told us that she had a very rare condition called **microtia**, which means that the ears don't form properly inside and out. He was nearly sure that Sophie had no ear canal, but further than that he couldn't tell us anything more, so he said he would refer her to the best person he knew to look after her. This was a consultant called Mr Trimble who had trained in Toronto, Canada and was at present working in Belfast. The specialist said the first thing to determine would be if Sophie could hear, and also to scan her head to assess the situation inside. He said it was likely that she would be fitted with a type of headband to enable her to hear by the conduction of sound through the bone behind her ears. She would eventually need surgery in a few years to drill out the canal and would probably have to go to Great Ormond Street Hospital in London. He handed Sophie back to Fiona and she broke down and cried. I took Sophie from her and I asked him if we should be optimistic and he said, "Oh yes, she will be able to hear." Colin shook his hand and thanked him as we left. Fiona was very upset and emotional and Colin and I were trying to console her. I remember Colin's words so well. He said, "She <u>will</u> hear us Fiona." Fiona said she was more upset because of what little Sophie would have to go through in the future. My wee daughter was finding this extremely difficult. Not only was she just getting over the birth of her first baby but she was having to deal with a situation that was tearing her to pieces - not easy when your hormones are all over the place. The pain was clear in Colin's face too and he was obviously trying to keep it together for Fiona. My heart was breaking for all three of them.

The appointment was made to see Mr Trimble at the Royal Victoria Hospital on Thursday 16th December. We were very impressed at the speed things were moving. So Fiona, Colin and Sophie had their first visit with a consultant who specialised in this field. He took all the usual details for his notes and then spoke about microtia. He said that it was a very rare congenital disorder which happened in one ear in 1:10.000 babies. It was even rarer to see it in two ears when it happened to 1:100,000 babies. There was no known reason as to why it should happen and it appeared to be random. Babies born with microtia may have no inner ear so he said there was a need to establish to what degree Sophie's ears were affected. He said she was too young at the moment for an MRI scan but hopefully in a couple of months that could be done. Mr Trimble said the important thing at the moment was for Sophie to have a hearing test to assess if she could hear. This would be carried out by placing electrodes on her head and measuring if there was any brain activity in response to a noise or sound. It was then discussed how Sophie could be helped and he explained the use of a BAHA (Bone Anchored Hearing Aid). This can be attached to a headband which she would wear with the hearing aid sitting on a bone. The idea is that all sounds are transmitted through the bone to the inner ear, if she has one. When asked about the future, Mr Trimble explained that in a few years she would probably have to have reconstructive surgery to build new ears, this would be carried out at Great Ormond Street or Birmingham Hospitals. He commented that Sophie had little ear lobes and added that many babies have very deformed ears, sometimes lower than usual, and in addition can have a misshaping of the face. He said he would arrange an appointment with the audiologist but as they were leaving the audiologist appeared and said there was time to do it then and there! This procedure involved placing electrodes to Sophie's forehead and behind her ears. Head phones were then placed next to her right ear and a high pitched sound was played, but there was no brain activity. However when the test was done by playing sound through the bone behind her ear there was brain activity. Sophie had responded to vibration behind her ears so that meant the sound had been conducted via the bone to her inner ear, proving that she definitely had working inner ears! The problem appeared to be restricted to the actual ear and the ear canal leading to the inner ear. It was then decided that the Baha was the answer for now and the earlier the better so she could hear sounds from an early age. So how can a child hear without a canal? The inner and outer ears form at a different time in utero. As a result the inner ear is usually perfectly normal and a specialised test can confirm this. As long as the inner ear is normal, sound does not need an outer ear or canal to reach it. Sound strikes the skull bone causing a very subtle vibration that reaches the inner ear. The inner ear then transmits a signal to the brain telling it that there is sound.

I remember I was doing some Christmas shopping in town that day and waiting for a call to let me know how the consultation went. When Colin phoned me and told me the good news I was over the moon. There was relief from everyone. We had been given hope that everything would work out in the long run. Yes there was a lot of work to be done and wee Sophie would have a tough time ahead, but with both sets of grandparents and close family always at hand there was no doubt that Sophie, Fiona and Colin would have all the support they needed. This was definitely going to be a better Christmas than anticipated!

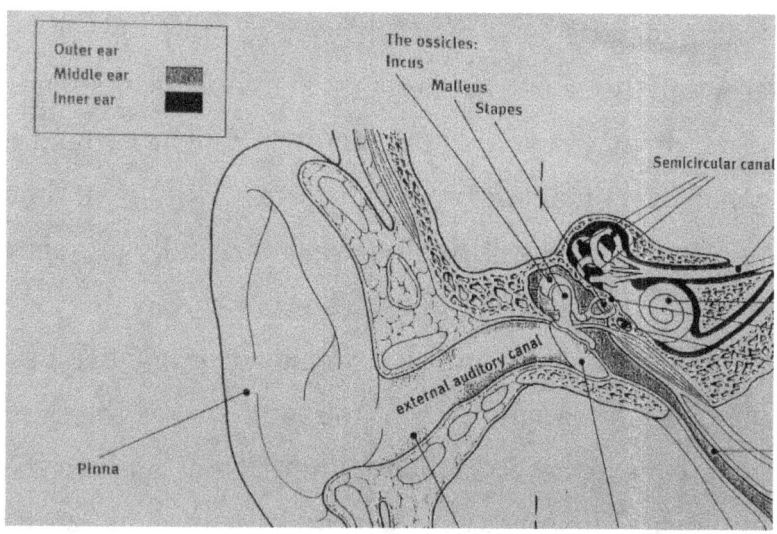

Figure 2: Diagram of ear and internal mechanisms

Chapter 2

The Early Months

We had a good Christmas with all the family and some good family days out at the beginning of January. The usual goodbyes were said to Melanie and Simon as they headed back to faraway places. I remember January 9th was a very quiet day after the buzz of Christmas and New Year and I felt a little low and of course from then on my mind was yet again on wee Sophie.

Mid-January I was feeling particularly low. I was waking up every morning thinking about Sophie. The excitement of Christmas was over, we had all been kept busy but now there was more time to think and I was struggling to get myself lifted. I was thinking about Fiona and if she was ok. She always seemed fine but I wondered if she really was coping or was she hiding her feelings from me. One morning I phoned Melanie in New Zealand. I told her how I was feeling and how worried I was about the development of Sophie's ears and her speech and what she would have to go through in the future. My daughter told me I shouldn't be worrying because everything was sorted and we knew what was going to happen. This really made me think. Yes things had settled and we had accepted them and had a good Christmas, but those feelings of sadness were still there deep down. It's not sorted, it's going to take a long time. It will be tough. We still don't know enough. I don't know enough and I want to know more. Questions are filling my head. Why is there no appointment yet to fit the headband? When it is fitted will Sophie hear anything? If Sophie can't hear normally will her speech be affected? When she eventually has the operations will she have full hearing? How will Fiona and Colin cope through all this?

It is funny how things affect your way of thinking. I

teach French to primary school children and I have got to know one of the teaching staff in a school I work in. Her daughter was expecting a baby around the same time as Fiona and she too had a lovely baby girl. It's very strange how we can feel in certain circumstances. In all honesty I didn't like how I felt when talking to this lady about her grandchild. I was picturing scenarios where it was the other way round. If it was the other way round and her grandchild was born with microtia I would probably be thinking thank goodness it didn't happen to Sophie. So is she thinking the same? Is she feeling sorry for me? If she is I know it's not in a bad way, she's probably relieved more than anything and she has a right to feel like that. But do I have a right to feel this way? Some people will say I don't. But I'm only human.

It's now nearing the end of January and after a dismal month, as it tends to be after Christmas, Sophie at last has an appointment on 25th January to be measured for her headband. The little headbands are cute and they have chosen three different ones in red, pink and beige. It was explained to Fiona and Colin that there will be one little earpiece attached which has to be placed on a bone. This can be behind the ear or on the forehead but Fiona has been advised to move it to a different place every 15 minutes because of the sensitivity of the bones at this early age. Of course Fiona and Colin are very curious about what Sophie will be able to hear so the nurse let them place it on their foreheads and plug their ears. They were amazed at what they were able to hear! They have to come back in two weeks to have the Baha (bone-anchored hearing aid) fitted and tuned to suit Sophie's hearing. This was a positive day when they felt something was being done. The nurse explained that Sophie would be wearing the Baha until she was about 3 years old when it would then be implanted behind the ear.

Fiona always visits me on Thursdays, it's our day together. Of course it's now Sophie and Fiona who visit! Some days we have plenty to occupy us and we don't talk about Sophie, but then there are days when I know we are both thinking deeply and find it hard to speak out. On one of those days Fiona was feeding Sophie and stroking her wee ears. I am looking at her and there are tears in her eyes as she says, "I love her so much mum and I feel so sad that this has happened to her. I just hope it wasn't anything we did wrong that caused it." She then tells me that she feels that other people appear to have forgotten so readily. It's as if the drama is over and Sophie will be alright in the end so 'what's the problem?' But as Fiona explains, it's not over. The worries are all there and there are plenty to come. How will she cope in school? How will other children treat her? How will she cope with wearing this Baha permanently and with the operations ahead? I told Fiona I felt exactly the same and had the same worries all the time. I was determined that when my daughter was upset and having a bad day, I wasn't going to be one of those mums who says 'Never worry it will be ok'. And so I cry with her and worry with her. We had a good chat and we promised always to be honest with each other about our feelings.

On 3rd February Fiona took Sophie to the family doctor for routine injections and a health check. The lady doctor said, "So this is Sophie Ross. I was told about her a few days ago. I had to look up what microtia was as I had never heard of it before." This confirms how little is known about the condition. She examined her ears, joints and tummy and then asked, "How soon did you realise she had a problem?" Fiona replied, "As soon as she was born and we saw her ears!" Then the doctor said, "It's amazing what can be done for deafness nowadays. Hopefully it won't be too long before she is able to sign!" This brought home to me the ignorance regarding microtia. When a doctor who has had to look up information on the condition, cannot understand that it is not labelled as 'deafness', what hope of understanding has any parent who is struggling to come to terms with its meaning. Yes, Sophie has a hearing loss but she is not deaf. In the next chapter I will discuss the meaning of the term microtia and how it affects different children in different ways.

It was 15th February and Fiona was at Amanda's husband's book launch. She had Sophie with her and she met many people who hadn't seen Sophie since she was born. A good friend of Amanda's just loved Sophie and thought she was gorgeous. Later she said to Amanda, "If you were ever to have a baby with deformed ears wouldn't you just pick ones like Sophie has because really her ears are the cutest ever!" I still laugh at this. It was an honest remark from someone who knew not to pretend everything was ok and had a great manner of expression. I know most people do not know what to say when they see Sophie's ears. They are afraid to ask what is wrong with them so they don't comment. Then there is always an awkwardness where you know that they have seen them, and they know that you know they have seen them and nobody wants to mention it!

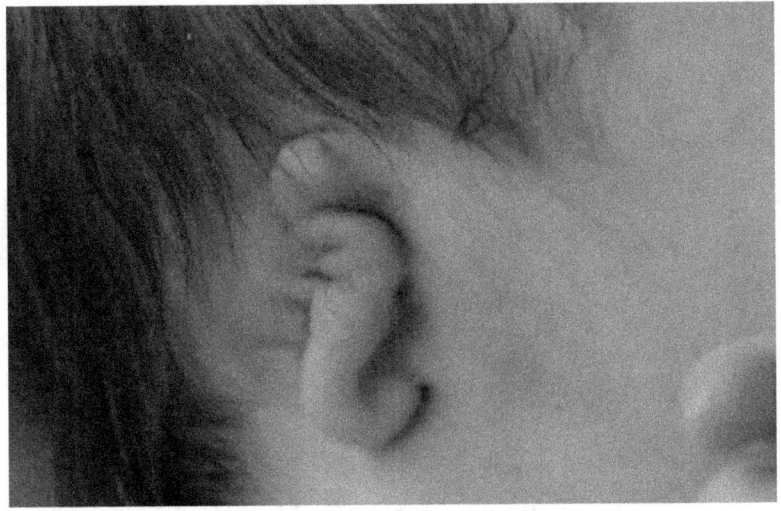

Figure 3: Sophie's right ear (both are the same)

So while waiting on the Baha fitting life goes on as normal! It was my birthday on 16th February. Fiona, Colin and Sophie took me out for afternoon tea. Sophie bought me a lovely mug and gave me a card. The next day I was out for afternoon tea again with Amanda, Noah and Megan and also Fiona and Sophie! Then we took Sophie to see our lovely neighbour Rosie who has loved Fiona since she saw her as a baby!

On another day we visited my mum who lives in Kilkeel, a little fishing town about 40 miles from

Belfast. My mum is almost 90 years old at this time and is a very wise lady. Of course she was delighted to see her little great-granddaughter and just loved nursing her on her knee. Fiona was out of the room when mum was chatting to Sophie on her knee. There is a way of talking to a baby as if the baby is talking to you, so with this in mind my mum says, "Great Granny, I have a tough struggle ahead of me, but I'll be ok, I'm a wee fighter!" This was a very poignant and emotional moment for me. I decided to leave it and tell Fiona on another day, as I was driving home and if I had said anything about it I would have cried!

In mid-February Fiona had a visit from a lady called Fionnuala McCreanor who is a Peripatetic Teacher of Hearing Impaired Children and works for the 'Service for the Sensory Impaired' who are based with the Southern Education and Library Board in Northern Ireland. The help and support that this organisation provides is explained in more detail in another chapter. Fionnuala admitted that she wasn't really aware of microtia and didn't know of many children with Bahas so she was very excited at the prospect of working with Sophie and also getting to know more about the condition. A support plan was drawn up with many targets. The details were very positive and carefully thought out. Concentration was mainly on the use of the Baha, making sure Fiona and Colin as parents know the role of the service provided, understanding Sophie's hearing levels and audiogram, knowing the general foundations of language, establishing hearing thresholds and discussing strategies towards development of her first words. All this is carried out with the liaison of home visits, ENT and Speech and Language Therapy. The visit was a great relief for Fiona and Colin, enforcing the idea that there is help out there from people who care.

Further to this, the day ended nicely with a call from Lorraine at the audio department of the Royal Victoria Hospital, to say she had an appointment for Sophie at 1.30 pm on 28th February to have her Baha fitted! Fiona was very excited and came off the phone shouting to Colin, "It's Monday for the Baha!" Then she promptly burst into tears as the emotions of the entire day caught up with her!

At this stage Fiona has mixed feelings about everything. She is excited about the Baha, but also worried. Finally getting the appointment makes everything more official and real. Up until now Sophie has been a good baby so you tend to forget about her ears! As the time draws near Fiona asks Colin if he is worried or scared about the appointment on Monday and he says he is actually alright about everything! Fiona finds this strange and wants to know how he can be so calm and not feel sad. He says he does sometimes when he really thinks about it but because she is such a happy baby he is happy. Fiona explains to him that she worries that she cannot really feel like that and always has mixed emotions and maybe there's something wrong with her, then Colin explains that he worries that he doesn't have mixed emotions and he wonders if there's something wrong with him! Fortunately the two of them end up having a good laugh about their different ways of thinking. The conversation is typical of a young couple who have been thrown into a different world with a new baby that has a rare medical condition.

And so the big day arrived, the day that Sophie would finally hear! It was explained to them that the earpiece would be set to the right ear only but that they could move it around the head. The audiologist showed them how to attach the earpiece to the headband and place it on a bone area. She warned them that Sophie would likely cry at her first sound, so she put it on and said, "Hello Sophie, can you hear me?" and Sophie subsequently burst into tears! Fiona found it very emotional and cried too, while Colin took Sophie and chatted to her. Then Sophie looked all round her and smiled. What a great and unforgettable moment for everyone!

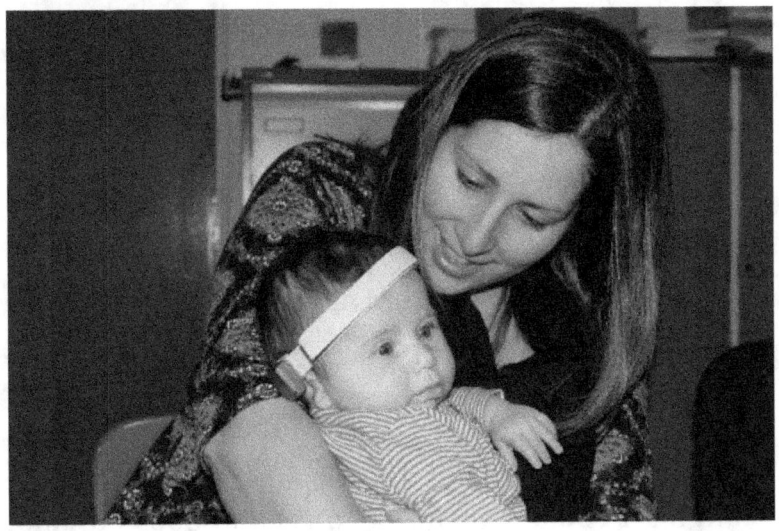

Figure 4: BAHA just fitted

The next step was an electrode hearing test. The guy in charge had Fiona, Colin and Sophie at one side of the room. He played different pitches of sound and Sophie looked around, but when it became too high she cried, so that was an indication that it was too loud.

Eventually the Baha was set to a level that wasn't too high and that would be it until an assessment on 13th May. At this stage the Baha was only to be worn for 15 minutes at a time and for about 3 times per day, and of course it was not to be worn during the night. Overall things had progressed and Sophie was now able to hear. Fiona and Colin were happy, even though Fiona thinks that the earpiece box sticks out further than she anticipated, however that's a small price to pay for the result!

I will always remember Sophie's first day out with her new Baha. It was 2nd March 2011 when Fiona and Colin took her to the park. Later that day I got a wee email from Sophie, alias Fiona!! It read:

"Hi Granny, I was at the park today and had my Baha on. I could hear all the girls and boys playing, the birds singing and also a big train that went past. It was really fun. I couldn't go on any of the play things as I am still a wee bit too small. I hope you like the pics of me and mummy. Love Sophie xoxo"

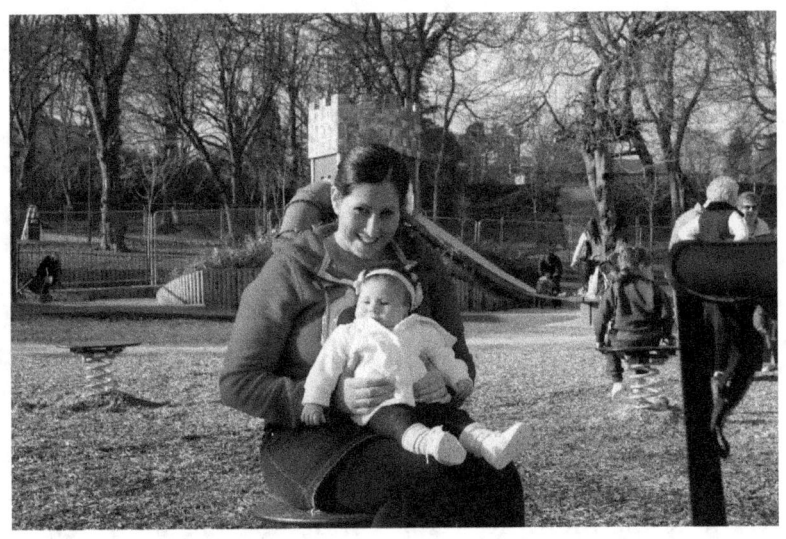

Figure 5: A moment to treasure for ever

There are good days mostly but there are days when we need to talk and express our feelings. There was an occasion when Fiona called me to tell me she had a moment when she got upset about Sophie's ears. She said while she had been feeding her she was watching her and was thinking how much she loved her. She felt heart-broken when she thought about what Sophie may have to go through in her life. It was one of those moments when we all feel that it is so unfair. Fiona knows Sophie is a happy little girl but it is the thought that she has no idea what is ahead of her. Fiona told me that deep down she knows that it will all be ok in the end but she still feels sad for her.

At the beginning of March Fiona had the opportunity of meeting a girl, Jennifer, who also has a child with microtia. Like Sophie, Rebekah has bilateral microtia but also has a cleft of her soft palette and one kidney. Getting to know another mum in the same situation as herself at this early stage has come as a blessing to both of them, especially as the two little girls are nearly the same age. As Fiona says it is great to know someone who really understands. Jennifer is convinced that little Rebekah was born at the same time as Sophie for a reason. I will come back to Rebekah's condition in the next chapter where I look into microtia.

Fionnuala came to visit again on 23rd March. She wanted to catch up on how Sophie was progressing. She said she would be referring Sophie to 'Speech & Language' and also would be contacting someone she knows from the 'National Deaf Children's Society'. Sophie is now wearing the Baha for 15 minutes, three times per day.

The second appointment with Mr Trimble was on 24th March. It was all normal hospital procedure with files piled high while listening for your name. When

Sophie is called in Mr Trimble is reading her file. He had to read the file to remember who Sophie was and said, "Ah Sophie from Lagan Valley hospital! Ok so how is she? Good?" Fiona replied with a short, "Yes she's fine," and he went on to say, "Ok so next is the fitting of the Baha." He had forgotten that she already had a Baha! Colin asked him when Sophie would be having a scan done and he said maybe around 1–2 years old. Mr Trimble made some reference to when Sophie would be a teenager and wearing her Baha, and Colin asked him what he meant. His reply was that that was in the future and there was no point worrying about it now. Easy to say but impossible to do. I would have hoped for more understanding and patience with a couple who are trying to come to terms with what has happened, but I do understand the pressure consultants are under.

Now it is April and the days are becoming longer and a bit brighter as spring tries to worm its way in! Mother's Day is late this year on 3rd April. Sophie got her mummy a mug with 'I Love Mummy' on it, a teddy and some bubble bath. They visited Colin's mum for a while then came to me. Unfortunately a couple of days later Sophie developed conjunctivitis and had to have some antibiotics.

Ronnie and I set off on 9th April to spend some time in our lovely house in France. This year was going to be very exciting as Fiona, Colin and Sophie were coming to stay with us for a week! Before that it was Fiona's birthday on the 12th and Sophie got her a cushion with 'Mum You're Perfect' on it. Sophie had her first overnight stay away in Dublin on the 15th when Fiona and Colin went with his mum and dad to celebrate his mum's 50th birthday. Sophie coped very well in a strange place!

Then on 19th April they all arrived in France. This was Sophie's first holiday and first time in an aeroplane. It was a lovely week, we had such a relaxing time and enjoyed every minute with our wee granddaughter! She was 4 months old then and very aware of her surroundings. She loved the outdoors, especially the trees. Every evening I carried her in my arms for a walk around the garden and she would look up at all the branches hanging down and reach up to try and touch them. She also loved the next door neighbour's collie called Tiny. She had no fear of anything and loved to watch Tiny running about. These were all very special moments to remember.

Sophie continued to develop like every child does,

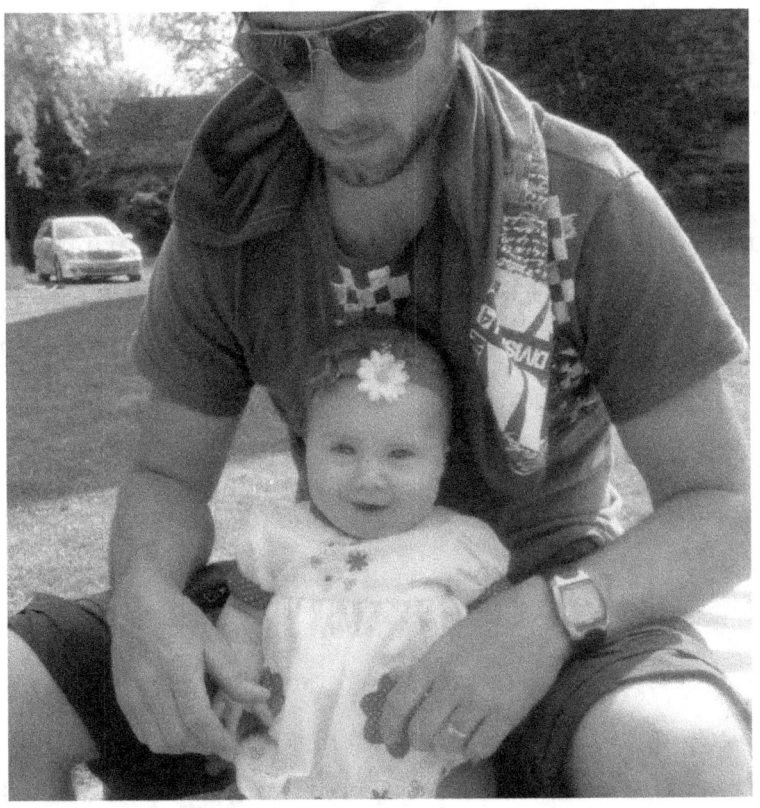

Figure 6: Sophie and her dad in France

having her first 'spoon-feed' on 29th April. Wearing the Baha just became a part of her life. It was obvious she could hear and she was a very happy child.

On 2nd May Colin's dad ran a Marathon in Belfast to raise money for a fund for Sophie. This was to help Fiona and Colin with any trips they might have to make in the future for Sophie's benefit. David was 54 years old then and found it quite exhausting. He was on the edge of giving up a few times but Colin pushed him on to the end and walked with him until he completed it! He raised £700 which was a great achievement!

In mid-May Sophie had her next audiology appointment with a girl from the SEELB 'Hearing and Impaired' department. The girl distracted Sophie by placing a toy on the table. Then the toy was hidden and she went behind her to make sounds and see if Sophie would turn round in response. However this didn't work as Sophie was only interested in finding out where the toy had gone! When the girl did come round to talk, Sophie did in fact turn her head towards her. It was decided that the test was inconclusive as she was too young to understand the concept of it, and it would have to be repeated in a couple of months. Then the girl in charge of the Bahas called in to see if the Baha needed adjusted. Nothing was done as the level appeared to be fine. Fiona was told that Sophie could now cope with wearing the Baha all the time during the day.

At this stage Fiona and Colin were given information to explain an audiogram. The following is an audiogram of familiar sounds.

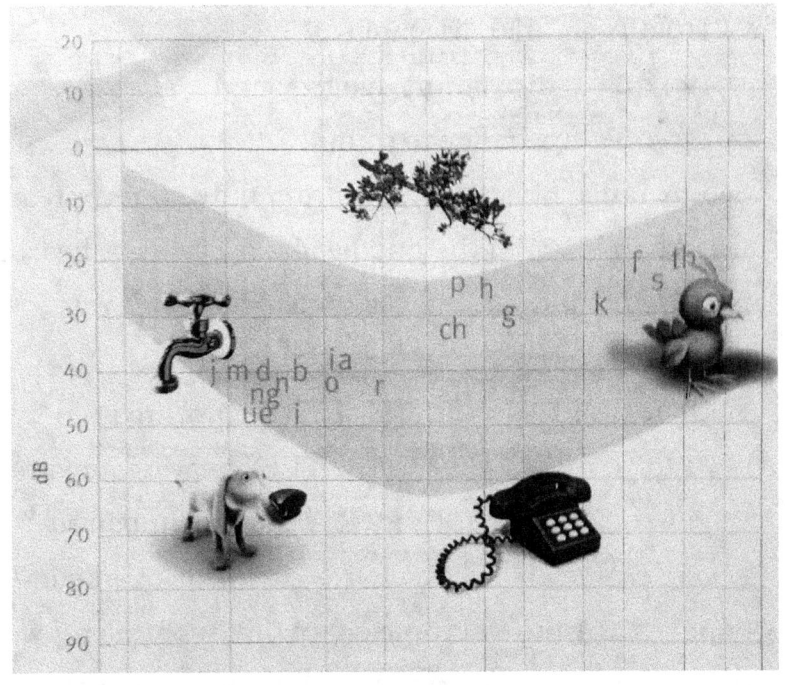

Figure 7: Audiogram

The hearing level is determined in decibels which relate to everyday sounds as follows:

    0 dB - the veritable pin drop
    20 dB - screening pass level for school testing
    40 dB - quietest speech you can discriminate
    60 dB - conversational speech
    80 dB - a shout
    90 dB - a loud shout

100 dB - a pneumatic drill
110 dB - loud disco music
120 dB - discomfort due to sound
130 dB - pain due to sound

So our range of hearing goes from 0 dB to 120 dB and we like to listen in the middle about 60 dB. A hearing impaired child has got a much reduced range of hearing as follows:

Up to 40 dB - SLIGHTLY hearing impaired
41 to 70 dB - MODERATELY hearing impaired
71 to 95 dB - SEVERELY hearing impaired
96 dB plus - PROFOUNDLY hearing impaired

Sophie's hearing test came out at 60 dB so this showed that she had a moderate hearing loss. At a push she could probably hear the phone ringing or a dog barking plus any louder sounds like an aeroplane, but she could not hear sounds like a tap dripping or a bird singing. The amplification from the child's hearing aid must go above this but stay below the child's thresholds of discomfort and pain.

Residual hearing is a term used to describe the hearing that remains after a hearing loss. This can be stimulated by amplifying sound using a hearing aid such as the Baha. As Sophie starts to communicate it will have to be determined if her residual hearing is low, high or across frequencies. Speech therapists will listen closely to her use of vowels and consonants in speech and determine the areas where there is help needed.

Next was a trip to the Health Centre to the Speech and Language Therapy department. They took a history and admitted they didn't know much about microtia either, so Fiona was able to enlighten them a bit on the subject! They performed different tests with maracas etc. and said Sophie's reactions were very good. They also gave Fiona an advice sheet on communication skills. It concentrates initially on trying to encourage a child's first words by choosing a word at a time to work on. This would involve a toy or activity that would encourage the use of this word and it was important that the child hear this word as many times as possible. From 6 months onwards it is very important to watch your baby to see how it responds to you. Fiona found all this information very useful and was determined to help Sophie's speech develop as naturally as possible and not let her fall behind just because she had microtia.

At the age of 6 months, Sophie was very well-travelled having just had her second holiday of the year in Majorca with her other set of grandparents! She was progressing well with the Baha and was developing like a normal 6 month old baby. Fiona and Colin were now able to see light at the end of the tunnel and had adapted to the situation very well.

On 27th July Sophie had to go and see a Geneticist in Belfast City Hospital. As there is no known cause for microtia, it is part of an ongoing search to look for links in children who have it. Apparently in the womb the kidneys form at the same time as the ears so it is vital to have some tests taken to see if there is a problem with the kidneys, as can be the case in some children. Sophie was given a thorough examination from head to toe. They looked for other facial abnormalities but were satisfied that all was well with her. She also had two normal functioning kidneys which was great news. So it appeared that Sophie's issue was isolated to the ears only, and also it was less likely to be a chromosome defect causing the microtia. They also said there were no guarantees that if they had another baby, it would not have microtia. Fiona told me later that it wouldn't really bother her that much if it happened again because she believed she could accept it better. I felt very content about this as I felt it conveyed her true acceptance of what had happened to Sophie.

Chapter 3

Microtia

I thought this would be a good time to look at the facts surrounding microtia. So what is microtia? When we were first told that Sophie had this condition we were completely in the dark. Of course we wanted to know all about it so I searched the Internet and tried to find out as much as possible. Yes I found a few things about it which did help, but what I was really looking for was a book that would tell us about it from all angles, what it is, what causes it, how it is treated, what is the long-term outlook, what can be done to help a child with it etc. So I looked for a book and found nothing with all the information I was looking for. This is what inspired me to write this book, I wanted something that future parents of children with microtia could turn to and find out everything they wanted to know, all in one place.

In this chapter I will explore microtia and the variations around it that affect every child differently. The next few paragraphs were put together at Great Ormond Street Hospital, London (GOSH), and will outline and describe the condition, from their perspective and experiences, in a very easily understood manner. Information has also been used courtesy of 'Children's Craniofacial Association' in Dallas, where it was put together voluntarily by healthcare professionals.

Microtia is a rare condition affecting about one in 7,000 babies. It seems to affect more boys than girls, and affects right ears more than left ears, although we don't yet understand why this should be the case. It also seems to be more common in Asian people than people of other races, but again we don't yet know why.

Microtia literally translated from the Greek means 'little ear'. It is the medical word to describe a small or absent ear. It is present from birth (congenital) and can appear on its own or alongside other symptoms as part of a syndrome. Some syndromes that have microtia as a feature include:

- Goldenhar syndrome
- Hemifacial macrosomia
- Treacher-Collins syndrome

If your child has microtia, does this mean that he or she is deaf in that ear? Most children with microtia will have some degree of hearing loss on the affected side. This is because the middle ear, which contains the eardrum and tiny ear bones, is affected as well as the outer ear. In some children, the ear canal is blocked or absent, so sound waves cannot pass through the ear in the normal way. Generally, although the outer and middle ears are affected, the inner ear is healthy, so some options for restoring hearing are available. Great Ormond Street Hospital do not recommend operations to repair the hearing tube and middle ear as they do not offer very good success rates, and in some circumstances could damage hearing further. This important subject will be addressed later.

Microtia can affect one ear only (unilateral) or both ears (bilateral). Children with unilateral microtia usually have normal hearing in their other ear, although this must be confirmed with hearing tests at a young age. Having normal hearing in only one ear will not usually result in any speech and language delay, and there are strategies to make the most of the child's hearing while at school, for instance. It is unusual for a child with unilateral microtia to need a hearing aid.

Children with bilateral microtia will usually need some form of hearing aid at a young age to enable them to develop speech. This is often a 'bone conduction hearing aid' that transmits sound waves to the inner ear through the bones of the skull. In very young children, these hearing aids are usually on a headband, but as a child grows older a 'bone anchored hearing aid' not on a softband but implanted, might be suggested.

Of course with Sophie, the first thing we wanted to know was if she could hear. A child with microtia often has a normal inner ear; therefore, in those cases children with microtia generally have some hearing in the affected ear. The presence of the ear canal and middle ear are variable. So, the amount of hearing also varies depending on the presence of these structures. If both of these structures are present, hearing in the affected ear can approach normal. It is important to note that if the opposite ear is unaffected, the child will have normal hearing in that ear, regardless of the condition of the affected ear. Since the inner ear is normal in the majority of children with microtia, those children with microtia on both sides still have the ability to hear. This type of hearing is often further enhanced with hearing aids to ensure normal speech and language development.

So how is microtia diagnosed? It will be obvious at birth that your child has a small or absent ear. Hearing tests will be used to work out whether your child has any hearing in the affected ear, and if so, to what degree. Your child's hearing in the unaffected ear will also be confirmed. This will be helpful in planning your child's education later in childhood. If the microtia is suspected as part of a syndrome, your child may need other tests to confirm or rule out the diagnosis. Some syndromes are inherited, in which case you may be offered genetic counselling.

So why is a child born with microtia? No one knows the real cause. It is not passed down in the family. The pregnancy itself is often uneventful. The chances of having a baby with microtia are about 1 in 7000. The cause may be related to poor blood supply to the tissue during ear development; however, this is only speculation. Since the causes are unknown, prevention is therefore difficult.

Finally does microtia affect normal development? Generally, having either one or two sided microtia does not affect development. This is true if early steps are taken within the first few months from birth to ensure that hearing is normal. These steps include seeing an ear, nose, and throat (ENT) surgeon, often a member of the craniofacial team, who can assess ear function and direct hearing aid placement if necessary. If the microtia is part of a syndrome, development may be affected depending on the syndrome and its severity.

The big question is, are there any treatments available? All the treatment options available in the UK are cosmetic. That is, they improve the look of the ear but cannot improve its function. There are three options for treatment available: no surgical treatment, ear construction using a rib graft and getting a false (prosthetic) ear. More information about each option follows. Your hospital team will discuss each option with you, and the final decision about which option to take will be made jointly between you, your child and the microtia team.

<u>No surgical treatment</u>: While your child is young, you

may decide to leave the ear as it is. Some children camouflage their ear by growing their hair long, while others deal with comments and questions more easily. If the child does not perceive having microtia as a problem both psychologically and emotionally, they may decide to leave things as they are. The chances of successful surgery or prosthesis improve with age, so if your child changes his or her mind in the future, these options will still be open.

Ear reconstruction using a rib graft: This involves making a new ear from your child's own tissue. The framework or 'scaffolding' is made from cartilage taken from your child's ribcage. The reconstruction is carried out in two stages. It is important that the cartilage is mature, so this option is not offered to children under ten years old. Most children are at secondary school when this option is offered. Advantages include the use of the patient's own tissue which means there is generally no rejection and there is a lower risk of infection. Disadvantages are that there is scarring left on the rib cage and skin grafting is required at the back of the ear.

False (prosthetic) ear: This involves attaching implants and fixtures to your child's head onto which a false ear is attached. This can be carried out on children around seven years old or more. It usually takes two operations: one to insert the implants and another to attach the fixtures. Once the operations are complete, the false ear is attached to the fixtures. The false ear itself is made from soft, silicone material and is sculpted to match your child's other ear. Advantages include an excellent colour match and a natural appearing ear and because there is only minor surgery involved, pain and scarring is minimal. Disadvantages include the need for replacements every two years and the fixtures need to be cleaned every day.

The decision for the best treatment method is something not to be taken lightly and should only be considered after discussions and meetings with your hospital team, family and most importantly, the child. The decision should uppermost meet the child's needs and desires i.e. social, emotional and psychological.

When should any treatment start? Theoretically, it would be best to treat children with microtia before they start school. However, there are various reasons why this is not possible. A child's ear reaches adult size around the age of six years, so treatment before this age could result in mismatched ears. If ear reconstruction is the preferred method, there is not enough cartilage in a child's body before the age of ten years.

As mentioned above, the surgeons in GOSH do not recommend surgery to repair the ear canal (this will become clearer in the next chapter). They believe that there are too many complications and dangers in this very delicate operation. It seems the most obvious and straightforward thing to do, but there are a lot of differences of opinion around it.

In the USA there are centres that offer the creation of an external opening and ear drum when relatively normal middle ear structures are present. The advantage of course is obtaining normal hearing in the affected ear. Disadvantages, however, include a variable success rate meaning that normal hearing may not be achieved after lengthy surgery. The new ear canal may also close, resulting in a scar in that area.

The absence of an external ear canal is referred to as aural atresia. When someone has aural atresia, there is a high incidence of malformation of the external ear and middle ear also, but the inner ear and auditory nerve are frequently normal. The big question for most parents is should they go down the road of trying to improve the hearing by this surgery. As I said above, atresia repair is carried out in the USA, but it is important to note that not all children with aural atresia are candidates. For them candidacy for atresia surgery is based on the hearing test (audiogram) and CT scan imaging. If a canal is built where one does not exist, minor complications can arise from the body's natural tendency to heal an open wound closed. Repairing aural atresia is a very detailed and complicated surgical procedure which requires an expert in atresia repair. While complications from this surgery can arise, the risk of complications is greatly reduced when using a highly experienced otologist. Atresia patients who opt for surgery will temporarily have the canal packed with gelatin sponge and silicone sheeting to prevent closure. The timing of ear canal reconstruction (canalplasty) depends on the type of external ear (microtia) repair desired by the patient and family.

After several years of experience with canal surgery first, followed by medpor as a second surgery, Dr Roberson, in cooperation with Dr John Reinisch, performed the first Combined Atresia Microtia Repair (CAM) surgery in the world in January 2008. The two doctors combined two previously separate fields of surgical practice into one unified surgery. This 8-9 hour outpatient procedure combines both the atresia repair canalplasty and the medpor outer ear reconstruction. At this time, they were the only ones in the world performing this surgery.

Commonly, in children with both sides affected, hearing aids are recommended to ensure normal hearing and speech and language development. There are two types of hearing aids: those that are worn on a headband and others that are anchored to the skull bone. You will see in the next chapter what Dr Reinisch, who works in Los Angeles, thinks of ear canal construction, compared with Mr Bulstrode (GOSH), both of whom Fiona, Colin and Sophie went to see in London in August 2011.

In the previous chapter I mentioned little Rebekah who also has microtia. Rebekah has bilateral microtia - right side grade 2 with ear canal and ear drum present, but a CT scan showed misformed ear bones, so conductive loss is the same as left side. Left side grade 3, ear lobe only and atresia.

Jennifer very kindly agreed to give me the following information about Rebekah, in her own words.

"Rebekah was born at 35 weeks, having a cleft of her soft pallet and not feeding so she was transferred to Neo Natal. It was during this time that we meet her consultant to be. He gave us no name for Rebekah's condition. My brother, Stephen, did some research online and came up with the word microtia and what grade she seemed to have. Rebekah was discharged from hospital without a new-born hearing screening and referred to RVH hospital. Rebekah was born on 11 July 2010 and we had to wait until 13 Oct for her appointment. During her first appointment with the Cleft Pallet Team sometime in August/Sept her Plastic Surgeon confirmed microtia and reassured us that he had numerous patients with microtia whom he referred to GOSH. Rebekah wears a headband with Baha bilateral BP110 currently on soft band with surgery planned late 15/early 16"

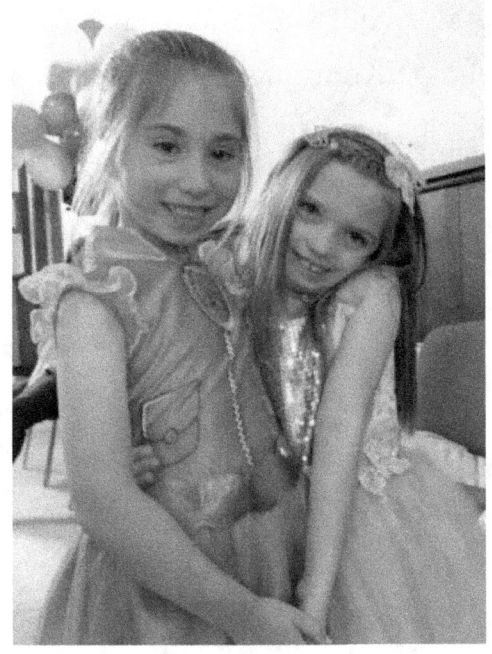

Figure 8: Rebekah's 7th birthday with Sophie age 6

On rare occasions microtia occurs with other abnormalities as part of a syndrome. The most common condition associated with microtia is 'hemifacial microsomia', in which half the face does not grow in proportion to the other. The degree of hemifacial microsomia varies from barely perceptible (most common) to very noticeable (less common). 'Treacher Collins Syndrome' involves both ears and also affects the eyes, which appear to have a downward slant or 'pulled down' appearance. The cheek bones are small and the eyelids and jaw are affected.

'Goldenhar Syndrome' may involve one or both ears and is characterised by incomplete development of ear, nose, soft palate, lip and jaw. These children often have abnormalities of the neck bones as well as a benign tumour of the eye. There are also other less common syndromes where microtia may occur.

What is everyday life with microtia really like? It can be hard to deal with looks or comments from strangers. The GOSH booklet 'Bringing up a child whose face looks different' was originally written for parents of children with birthmarks but contains plenty of strategies for dealing with any unwanted comments or attention. It was written by one of their psychologists with many suggestions from parents. Parents have said that it can be difficult to know how to help a child who has hearing in one ear only. There are various strategies you can use at home and discuss with your child's school.

At home your child will find it easier to hear you if you stand or sit on the side of their hearing ear. This is especially important if there is background noise from the television or brothers and sisters. If you suspect your child has an ear infection in the hearing ear, visit your family doctor (GP) promptly. At school ask if your child can sit towards the front, with his or her hearing ear near the teacher. Learning to read may be more difficult if certain sounds are difficult to hear over classroom noise. Ask if quiet reading time is possible on the timetable. Check your child's eyesight regularly so that he or she can read instructions easily. Talk to the Special Educational Needs Coordinator (SENCo) about any other aids that might help your child.

What is the outlook for children with microtia? As discussed in the treatments section, operations carried out in the UK to correct microtia will only make the ear look better. It will not improve how well it works. The results from surgery are usually very realistic and will rarely need repeating in later life. The majority of children adapt to any hearing loss, growing up to work, study and have children. The child will live with having microtia and the consequences of its treatment his or her entire life. Therefore, it cannot be overstated that the principles of treatment for facial appearance should be guided by the child. Surgery or prosthesis fitting generally occurs between 6 and 10 years of age. This timing varies, depending upon how the child is coping socially and psychologically and also on the growth of the face and body.

One thing always on my mind was if microtia would affect Sophie psychologically. This is a complex question and as well all children cope differently depending on their personalities. Having microtia may not affect your child at all or it may affect self-esteem, body image perception and confidence. This depends on multiple factors including family interactions, family and child education about microtia, the school environment and whether your child has developed or been taught the tools to cope with his or her differences. The social worker and child psychologist that are a part of the craniofacial team are a good resource for starting the education process. They can help with opening the avenues of communication between family members and even coordinating meetings between families who have already gone through the treatment process. These families can often be important resources for information, offering real-life experiences to families just beginning the treatment process.

Chapter 4

Meeting Surgeons

In April 2011 Fiona's friend Jennifer sent her a copy of an article explaining that surgery using something called 'medpor' was available in Australia and the USA. Fiona did some research and found that it was carried out by a Dr Reinisch from the 'Cedars-Sinai Center for International Health' in Los Angeles. She got things moving by sending emails and making inquiries about their treatment for children with microtia and by a stroke of luck it emerged that Dr Reinisch would be coming to London in August of this year and would be happy to meet with them, if it could be arranged, for a free consultation! Well, if you are going to London why not make the travel worthwhile and see if you can meet with someone from Great Ormond Street Hospital at the same time! This is exactly what Fiona did and managed to make an appointment to see Mr. Neil Bulstrode, Consultant Plastic and Reconstructive Surgeon at GOSH. Unfortunately this private appointment was going to cost them £230 for 20 minutes of his time. However both visits were arranged to take place within a day of each other! And so on 1st August 2011 Fiona, Colin and Sophie set off for London to visit these two very experienced and competent surgeons. My hope was that surely they would come back with some great news. I was already thinking of ways we could all work together to raise enough money to take Sophie to the USA if that was where the solution lay. I was excited about this trip they were making because they needed answers and so did I. We needed reassurance that there was something out there to help our little Sophie.

Dr John Reinisch MD is one of world's leading paediatric plastic surgeons and an innovator in his field. He is currently Director of Craniofacial and Pediatric Plastic Surgery at Cedars-Sinai Medical

Center in Los Angeles. He is a world-renowned paediatric plastic surgeon and a pioneer in the field, having developed the medpor method of ear reconstruction for treatment of microtia. He founded the division of plastic surgery at Children's Hospital Los Angeles in 1983 and was also chairman of the division of plastic surgery at the University of Southern California, where he remains on the faculty.

Traditionally, plastic surgeons have relied on a technique that removes cartilage from the patient's rib and uses it to rebuild the ear. Reinisch believes that this method, though effective, has two major limitations: it requires a large number of surgeries to complete and also cannot be performed until a child is 10 or 12 years old and at the age where they have a large enough quantity of rib cartilage. By this time, he believes that the effects of living with a deformity have often taken a toll on the child emotionally. And so he envisioned a new technique that would save children and their families the discomfort of multiple surgeries and the emotional pain a facial deformity can cause.

His pioneering work in medpor ear construction surgery has helped and transformed the lives of thousands of children with microtia. The 'Reinisch' technique of medpor surgery is a one-time procedure with no hospitalisation, no scar and minimal pain. It can be done at around 3-4 years before nursery age to help children with microtia attain mental and emotional well-being. Before I look at this in detail, below are the details of the meeting. This is a summary of what was discussed, using his own terminology.

Dr Reinisch very warmly welcomed Fiona and her family into his sister's home in London where he was staying for a few days and meeting with some children he had helped through surgery. Initially he addressed the fact that some children have unilateral hearing and some bilateral. In Sophie's case of having bilateral microtia, he said something had to be done about the hearing. Also there's debate about unilateral hearing loss in terms of localising sound and hearing in a noisy environment with sound only coming in through one ear. He said that without the Baha Sophie would not develop language very well. He went on to explain how there is the outer ear, the middle ear and the inner ear. Most children with microtia have a normal inner ear, so they can still hear a lot of sounds. Sound vibrates the bone and the bone vibrates the middle ear.

Usually they can hear 60-70 db, anything less they

can't. Speech is 40 db, so they won't hear speech or whispers, but loud sounds yes. Fiona informed him that when Sophie was tested she could hear 60db. He then explained to them that the option is to make a canal, which is dependent on how good the middle ear is, but you cannot determine that until the child is about 2 and a half years old. At that stage they would have to have a CT scan. The radiologist, he said, will read it and write notes that will mean very little to anyone outside of the medical profession! The results will then go to the surgeon to see if he can work with the bones. If the bones are fused, or not connected, the sound coming in will vibrate to the eardrum but the bones will not move and do their job properly and therefore not produce the sound. This is the main factor determining whether or not you can have a new canal. So he said the first step Fiona and Colin need to take is to find out if Sophie is a candidate for a canal, and if she is, then ask themselves if it is what they want to do. He agrees that some people on the other hand would say no as you can just alternatively still wear a Baha, especially being a girl!

Dr Reinisch went on to explain that the Baha implant system is one that transmits sound vibrations through to the skull bone and to the inner ear. It will go to both sides so you can tell the sound direction. He then explained something else called the 'sound bridge system' and a new kind of Baha called the 'sophono', where you don't have to have anything protruding through the skin. There is a magnetic plate implanted and a device with a magnet on the outside that goes on the skin and it vibrates through the skin. This new system has just been approved. Otherwise with the bone induction implant you have a hole through the skin. He pointed out that although there can be some issues with that, they can be dealt with. The difference is that the sophono Baha vibrates through the skin but loses some vibration getting through to the bone. Dr Reinisch believes it is better having sound going right to the bone in order to have a better quality of hearing. The discussion went on to the subject of making a prosthetic ear. He explained to them how silicone was used for people with cancer who lost their nose and were unable to wear glasses. With silicone you can get the colour to match the face but the disadvantage is you have to put it on and off and also you have to change it as they do not last a lifetime and will fade with time.

According to Dr Reinisch there are two ways of

making the ear, using either rib cartilage or medpor. He explained how you can take a piece of rib cartilage when the child is 7 years or older, depending on the child's frame and development. But ideally you should wait until a child is 10 years old because they say if you take a large amount of cartilage from the chest earlier it can leave a deformity. The cartilage is carved and slipped underneath the scalp so you are lifting up the scalp and putting it underneath. Unfortunately if you have a hairline there you will end up having an ear with hair on it. This technique has been around since 1959. He describes how he has seen that ears made with cartilage can be a problem. Firstly taking a lot of cartilage from the rib can cause a deformity. Then because children have to wait until they are 10 years old to have this procedure, they are more aware they are different from other children, so it is best having something you can do when they are younger.

This led him on to putting forward his confidence in the use of medpor which was first introduced by himself in 1991. Medpor ear reconstruction is a surgical technique used for microtia patients that uses a synthetic framework and the body's tissue to create an ear. Dr Reinisch is a leader in this ear reconstruction technique.

Reconstruction with the medpor technique can usually begin around age three. If only one ear is involved, the medpor framework is customised to match the normal ear, but is created slightly larger in younger children so the ear will be adult-sized. The framework is then covered by the patient's own tissue (called a flap) which is brought down as a thin 'living membrane' from underneath the scalp. In most cases, a second surgery may be required to refine the reconstructed ear.

Dr Reinisch has further developed the medpor technique to significantly decrease scarring and achieve better results, including less chance of permanent hair loss. This approach enables them to harvest the 'living membrane' flap without any incisions on the scalp, hiding the scar behind the new ear. The flap is often covered with better coloured skin from the head, which usually leaves no scar.

Recently introduced into their practice is a combined one-stage reconstruction for both microtia and atresia using medpor. This advance offers a child with bilateral microtia/atresia to have completely functional and aesthetic reconstruction of both ears in three outpatient surgeries before the age of four.

Dr Reinisch explained to Fiona and Colin how this substance is porous, so tissue actually grows through the implant after a few months. He described how it is made and how it can be carved and made smaller or bigger as required. It is covered with a very thin layer of tissue such that if it was held up you would be able to see the blood vessels through it. This in turn shrinks around it, the air is then sucked out and then skin put on it. He emphasised that you cannot put skin on plastic, but with medpor, because you have a living membrane over the plastic, you then can put skin on. He said it will normally last a long time but conceded that they have had occasions where they had broken. The oldest one was made 20 years ago. When done it is protected with a cup for the first 3 weeks, then a silicone 'huggy' for night time for about 3 months. He says that if he does it for anyone outside of the USA he encourages you to take photos and send them to him so he can gauge how it is doing and subsequently give advice.

Fiona asked him about drilling out a new canal. Dr Reinisch said that it is unusual for a doctor to make a canal because it is a speciality and only really experienced surgeons will do it. Sometimes, because they have to deal with all kinds of issues, not many are done. He said there are a lot of things to look out for, for example a thing called a colestiatoma, where sometimes when the ear is forming, a little piece of skin can form and doesn't have a way to get out and consequently a cyst develops. But he said it is 2 years 6 months before you can tell this from an x-ray. If the x-ray shows this then sometimes a canal can be made just to get the cyst out and then you get the hearing at the same time. He said that where he lives in Los Angeles they have a place called the 'House of the Ear Institute' named after founder John House, where the cochlear implant was developed. They only do 10-12 canals a year so it is not a very common surgery. But Dr Reinisch said he has worked with a doctor who does 80-90 a year. He says these doctors just get better and faster at doing it. Fiona asked if the canal is drilled out before the ear construction. He explained that there are two ways to do it. They are both relatively short surgeries taking about 2 hours. But you do not carry out the two procedures at the same time because if you injure the nerve the Baha will not work either. You have to make sure the nerve is ok. When a hole is being drilled in the bone the bone vibrates and that energy can damage the nerve. He said they have had injuries, not big ones, but enough to drop the frequency of surgery. When they drill down to being almost there they stop and do the last part with a laser which doesn't cause any vibration. So that is one option, you drill the canal first and hopefully you hear and do not have to use the Baha. Then you make the ear. Dr Reinisch told how he did three the previous week. He had a boy from China and did the canal and the ear on Tuesday and Wednesday. On Thursday he had a boy from Dubai who was not a candidate for a canal but he was quite happy with how he approached it. He admitted that surgeons do not always get off with one surgery, sometimes you have to come back. When doing the ear, he said they do not put drains in anymore. They used to put suction in for two days but the patients could not cope when it came out, so now they put a dressing on that they try to keep on for two weeks. The patient comes back and the dressing is taken off and everything is well cleaned. A cup is put on so that the child cannot roll over when sleeping as it is important that they do not lean on that ear. So the ear can be done and not the canal, therefore a Baha is worn instead. He said that in his country the Baha (the screw in one) is not approved until the child is aged 5 years as the bone is not really thick enough. Another reason is that in younger children it can be put in too close to the new ear. They prefer to wait until the child grows a bit and then screw it in back from the ear a bit as it pivots and they do not want it touching the ear.

Dr Reinisch went on to point out that with cartilage you cannot make the canal until after the cartilage ear is done, but with him if you have a canal done they can make the medpor ear round it. He was very excited about this procedure as they had a girl with bilateral microtia and they made the canals when she was 3 years old and the ears a year later.

He stressed that the big issue was feeling when it was right to make a canal. As the canal is made first before the medpor ear, it is necessary to firstly have a cat scan to see if you are a candidate for a canal, if not you can just have the ear made, this is called atresia repair. The canal can be done separately or as combined surgery. He showed Fiona and Colin a lot of photos of different cases. So what are the costs involved? Obviously it is cheaper to do the ear only. Dr Reinisch explained that it is $30,000 for ear surgery and that involves the surgeon, operating theatre and anaesthetist. Combined surgery for canal and ear is about $70,000. If the surgery is carried out separately, that is the canal first then the new ear at a later date, it is about $10,000-15,000 more. The important question for Colin was if it was better in the long run to get the canal done if at all possible. Dr Reinisch stressed that the Baha was the most consistent form of hearing but there are disadvantages like taking it off when swimming etc. He said a child can get good hearing when the canal is drilled out but that depends on the circumstances surrounding the issue. He unashamedly said that if your child is 6 or 7 years old and the difference in cost between having the canal drilled out and using a Baha is $30,000 then he would just advise to put the money into a college fund and just use the Baha! So in the long run for cosmetic purposes the ear will cost $30,000. He admitted that drilling the canal does not always work for many reasons. There can be damage done to the drum. Also the canal will need to be cleaned out every 3 months as there are skin grafts inside and the dead skin has to be removed. There is a risk of infection too. In addition hearing is not always attained to the level wanted because it is not a perfectly normal canal. And if you have two microtic ears you can only drill one canal at a time so you would have to go home and return for the second one. He said the new canal does not produce wax but there is no problem with water getting in them.

Microtia is not very common, and varies greatly by the location of the culture. It is unilateral 90% of the time and is mostly on the right and more common in boys than girls. In fact 60% boys and 60% on the right. What causes it, we do not know, it does not seem to run in families, it just happens. In America there was a study where they tried to find twins that were identical and twins that were fraternal that had microtia. They found about 35 sets. So in non-identical twins they looked at how common one-sided microtia was in their group, and there was only one case where both of the twins had it. It was presumed that they had the same environmental factors. Then they looked at identical twins who genetically have the same material and there were 10 sets who both had it, so it seems like there is some genetic tendency to having microtia. On the other hand if it were that simple they would all have it, so it is really not that clear. Here is a description of how the ears tend to look in the different grades of microtia.

Grade 1 microtia: The ear is smaller than normal although most of the features of a normal ear such as a well-defined lobule, helix and anti-helix are present. This can occur with or without an external auditory canal.

Grade 2 microtia: The normal features of the ear are missing. There is still a lobule and a remnant of helix and antihelix.

Grade 3 microtia: 'The Classic Microtia'. The ear consists of a vertical skin appendage with a malformed lobule (earlobe) on the lower end. There is usually firm tissue at the upper end which is made up of a disorganised cartilaginous vestige. The lower end is usually a piece of lobular tissue which will be the future earlobe when reconstructed. Usually there is no external auditory canal (atresia).

Grade 4 microtia: No ear. This ear deformity, the most severe form of microtia, may at times be called anotia.

Sophie has Grade 3 microtia.

Neil Bulstrode is a Consultant Plastic Surgeon at Great Ormond Street Hospital for children and is the Lead Clinician for the Plastic Surgery Department. He is at the forefront of all new procedures and techniques. This involves the reconstruction of genetically deformed children, ear construction, craniofacial surgery, the treatment of giant congenital naevii (moles) and vascular anomalies. "Plastic surgery is my passion. It is important to appreciate and use the powerful techniques used in reconstructive surgery to improve the results of cosmetic procedures, and to use my cosmetic surgical skills to enhance the results of plastic and reconstructive surgery."

In the meeting with Fiona, Colin and Sophie, Mr Bulstrode asked how Sophie was affected. Apart from the fact that she had little ears he wanted to know if there was anything else wrong with her. They said that there was nothing that they knew of but arrangements had been made for her to have other tests on her kidneys, spine etc. He asked if anyone else in the family had small ears and if Fiona's pregnancy had been normal. He was satisfied no one else had the condition and her pregnancy had gone well. He said Sophie was obviously fine and looked perfect!

Mr Bulstrode went on to explain how he made ears for children who were born with little ears, and said he had actually made a couple that very day! He made it clear that they do not make the ears until the children are about 9 or 10 years old and said that was for a number of reasons. Firstly it was best to wait until then so that the patient would have an adult sized ear. He explained how at the moment they take the rib cartilage to create and carve and make the frame and that they have to take quite a bit of rib. Also he reconstructs the rib margins to minimise defect in the chest. The framework is then carved and put into a pocket of skin.

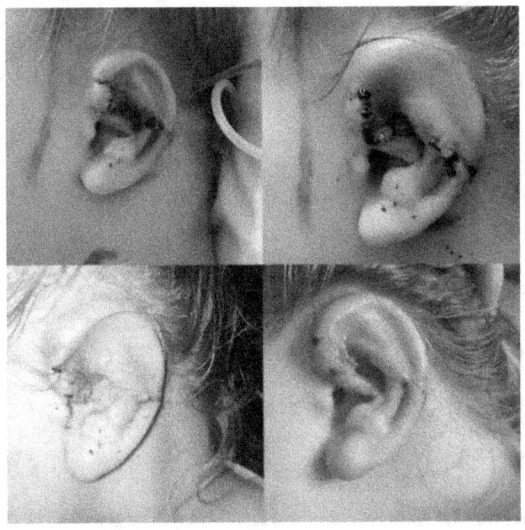

Figure 9: A first stage ear reconstruction by Mr Bulstrode

Then Fiona asked him the big question. "What do you do about the canal?" He said the canal was a different issue. People have historically tried to build canals but there has not been a great improvement in how they actually hear. He pointed out that if someone operates in this area before he gets to do his bit it really restricts his options in making a really nice ear. He said he needs to be able to operate on a virginal area, as it means he can make an ear as nice as possible. He agreed that logically you would think that if a canal was made it would help the hearing, but it does not work like that. In the surgery involved to drill out the canal, the hole that has been made often scrunches back down, with multiple infections, and it does not improve the hearing enough to warrant its worth. He clarified that with microtia the ear is made up only of the outer ear, which is slightly deformed, and the hole is not there. The middle ear is where the drum joins up to these little bones. The inner ear is where the 'snail' is for the balance, sound and all the little bits and bobs. He told them that it was likely Sophie's inner ear was normal, but in her case the middle ear was probably slightly deformed as the bones are slightly off. So if you did make both a canal and a drum, which is a very difficult thing to make, they would not move as well. For Sophie right now it is like putting your finger in your ear. That is how she hears, a sort of muffled sound. That is why she has this bone conduction hearing aid.

Fiona really needed to understand about the ear canal so she then asked him if he constructed the ear first and then do the canal after. Then the bombshell came..... This is the actual conversation that took place as it is of great significance to Fiona and Colin.

Mr B: "Well the thing is we don't make canals at all."

Fiona: "You don't make canals?"

Mr B: "No because it doesn't improve the hearing."

Fiona: "You don't drill a hole at all?"

Mr B: "Do you mean to look like a hole?"

Fiona: "Well yes but both...."

Mr B: "Well can you see my canal?"

Fiona: "No."

Mr B: "Right, you would have to look right in to see a canal."

(Shows them the ear he made today).

Mr B: "You don't actually need a hole to make it look like an ear."

(Shows framework he carved from rib, how shadow

makes it look like there's a hole there).

Fiona: "I just don't understand how it wouldn't improve her hearing if it was opened up and her inner ear was ok."

Mr B: "Well logically you would think that would be the case and people have done that in the past but it hasn't worked."

Colin: "Has it never worked?"

Mr B: "Not enough for the ENT surgeons here to think that it's a good idea."

Fiona: "So she will just have to wear a hearing aid for the rest of her life really?"

Colin: "We didn't know that, we were told that they would be able to drill through."

Mr B: "Who told you that?"

Fiona: "Well a specialist at home said the canal could be opened up and she then wouldn't need the hearing aid."

Mr B: "Has she been scanned?"

Fiona: "No".

Mr B: "Well.....my colleagues and I all agree it's not worth it. Maybe things will change in the next 5 or 10 years. We are also researching into how we can grow cartilage so we don't have to take the ribs. So these are the things we are trying to push ahead and who knows those options may be a possibility later. I'm sorry to disappoint you with this."

Colin: "It's ok. I just think the priority is for her to hear the best and properly."

Mr B: "Yes the hearing is the number one priority for her education, her speech and her communication."

This conversation was the one that changed everything for Fiona and Colin. They had finally been told straight out that re-building the canal was really not an option. This was much different than the way Dr Reinisch in the USA approached things.

Mr Bulstrode went on to explain how the preference for him and his colleagues is to put a Baha in place which must be placed 6 or 7 cms back from the ideal position of where the opening would have been to give enough room to make the ear. He said they would not do that until the age of 4 or 5 years perhaps. Fiona wanted to know if Sophie would need one or two hearing aids. Mr Bulstrode said ideas on that were changing. It was mostly one and now people were wondering whether to get two for slightly better hearing. He then stressed that the Baha is not without complications. The metal stud that comes through the skin often has infection there which has to be treated. The thing to remember is that your surgeon has to put it far enough back for the reconstruction. Fiona went on to tell him about their appointment with Dr Reinisch, the American doctor. She asked Mr Bulstrode his opinion on medpor. His response was that he would not use anything synthetic other than tissues from the body so that when it heals, it heals as part of the person. He said there was a high rate of infection if you get any exposure of the medpor and then it has to come out. He emphasised that if the ears he makes become infected they can be treated and will heal as they are living tissue and part of the body.

When asked which ear looked better he said that with his way you can carve a framework to match the other ear where you cannot do a framework with medpor.

Mr Bulstrode said that he does not believe in complicating things by using difficult procedures. He can discharge people after 6 months and they only come back if they have a problem, whereas with deeper procedures it requires going back, fixing, redoing and putting the child through a lot unnecessarily. His operations are in two stages but on both ears at the same time. Colin asked him why do a scan if they are not going to drill a hole. He said the only reason he can see for doing a scan would be to assess the thickness of bones etc. for the Baha but he himself would not do a scan unless he was going to use it for something in the future, because it is a big dose of radiation. For him a CT scan is not going to change what he is going to do. However he did say that Sophie may well need it if she is getting a bone anchored hearing aid put in. He made a point that in the NHS he personally does not have a financial drive to do anything quickly or before its time, he does it when he thinks it is best, whereas in the USA there is a financial goal. Colin explained that when Sophie was born they were told quite quickly that her canals would be drilled out and she would hear as normal, so really they wanted to get as much information as possible, and it is now disappointing to hear the real truth. Mr Bulstrode was very sympathetic and apologised for this but told them they are in no rush for decisions. He said that Sophie may not even want new ears and with long hair her ears would not be noticeable. He commented that she had no other disfigurements, her face was normal and her jawline and her ear positions were the same, so she had no noticeable abnormalities as such. This is very rare in bilateral microtia - "Her particular bilateral microtia is a rare thing because there are normally other complications associated with this disorder." This was really good to hear and very much to Sophie's advantage.

So here we have two meetings with two surgeons who do things differently. One process could involve making new ear canals and new ears in the USA for thousands of dollars but is the outcome certain and without problems? Is it going to be worth it in the end to put Sophie and her parents through long distance travelling, worry and pain to have procedures carried out in another country while being unsure of the outcome? In spite of all this should Sophie be given that chance? Or is it better to leave well alone and go with the bone implanted Bahas?

After this there was a lot of thinking to do, but no matter what, the decisions have to be the best thing for Sophie and her future. She is what matters most.

Chapter 5

Help!

When your child is born with any type of condition, the worst feeling is being alone and isolated. For most parents the condition is clear from the child's birth, and already, when you are supposed to be enjoying the birth of your baby, a fear of the unknown sets in. I know that my mind was conjuring up all kinds of problems and fears as soon as I knew that Sophie had a problem with her ears. Is she deaf? Will she ever be able to hear? How will Fiona and Colin cope? Why did this happen to my gorgeous daughter's first baby? The questions are endless and there are just no immediate answers. The first few days are spent asking questions, seeing doctors and specialists and frankly ending up confused when you hear different explanations from different people. Finally you go home with this little bundle not knowing what the future holds for it or your family and asking who, apart from your family, is going to help you through it. It is very scary!

Well, believe me there is a lot of help out there and I have been amazed at how many organisations and services are there for support. I know there will be different levels of support depending on where you live but if you feel you are not getting enough help, you must ask for it. Fiona has been very fortunate from the onset and has always had someone to turn to when she needed help and advice, and fortunately the help is still there and will be for as long as she needs it. I want to share some of this with you in the hope that if you feel you are not getting enough support, this will encourage you to seek advice from the right people.

After Sophie's birth Fiona and Colin met with and spoke to a few people, and it was evident that some of them did not really know much about microtia. However, at that stage you want to cling on to anything that sounds hopeful. If someone said that Sophie would be able to hear, you really want to believe that, but when someone says it is doubtful if Sophie will ever hear then you want to get someone else's opinion on it. There was a lot of confusing information for us at the beginning so my advice, with hindsight, is to listen to everyone carefully and be realistic until you get proper help with the right organisations.

Of course the main support comes from your consultant and the audiology department at your hospital. If you have a child with a permanent or partial hearing loss and who uses hearing aids, you will need to attend your community and/or hospital audiology clinics regularly during pre-school and school years. Regular appointments with Sophie's consultant Mr Trimble and Lorraine from audiology gave Fiona and Colin that feeling of security and care where they were assured everything was being done to help. A profile with details about Sophie's condition was built up, full of information on her hearing loss and her treatment. You may not agree with them all the time, but that is what they are there for, to answer any queries and doubts you may have! There will be times when you will have to visit the hospital for hearing aid repairs, or in

Sophie's case, when her hearing aid was lost! Having the same people, like Lorraine, is a consistency that I feel is very important. She has known Sophie since birth and has tested her regularly throughout the first few years of Sophie's life, not forgetting the fitting of the Baha and later on the support after the fitting of the bilateral implants. It is also important for Sophie too to see that familiar face on a regular basis.

As mentioned previously, one of the first people Fiona got home support from was a lady called Fionnuala McCreanor who is a 'Peripatetic Teacher of Hearing Impaired Children' and works for the 'Service for the Sensory Impaired' that is based with the Southern Education and Library Board in Northern Ireland. Fionnuala, who had not been aware of microtia until she met Sophie, has been, and still is amazing in the work that she does. She has loved the learning curve working with a child with microtia and in doing so was able to apply her experience and knowledge of working with the deaf and partially deaf. She has helped Fiona and Colin through rough times and has always been there when needed. The service provides a comprehensive programme of support to children with hearing and/or visual impairments and to their schools, parents, carers and supporting professionals. The programme includes hearing and vision assessments and advice on the children's needs, pre-school support, specialist teaching support for children attending school and provision of resources and adaptations where necessary. All the services are provided wherever children are and whenever their teachers, carers and support staff require it. This includes the home, playgroups, nurseries, nursery schools and mainstream and special schools. The majority of children with hearing or vision difficulties are identified at the pre-school stage and support commences at this time. Diagnosis is traumatic and families are given a significant amount of home-based support at this time. The support is extensive and includes peripatetic support (in class and withdrawal from), intensive language support for hearing impaired children, support to families and carers, acting as an advocate for children and young people, promoting inclusion for all, provision of audiological services, assessment and monitoring of children's developmental needs and the provision, evaluation, monitoring and maintenance of specialist equipment in schools.

Fionnuala's support is ongoing throughout playgroup and nursery years as you will see when we examine Sophie's progress later on. The service this organisation provides is exceptional.

Another very important source of help is the Speech and Language Therapy Department of your hospital. Speech and Language therapists (SLTs) are allied health professionals. They work closely with parents, carers and other professionals, such as teachers, nurses, occupational therapists and doctors. There are around 14,000 practicing SLTs in the UK. You should automatically be referred to them when your child is 6-12 months old. Communication difficulties put children at greater risk of poor literacy, mental health issues and poorer employment outcomes in adulthood. Speech and Language therapy is a vital service that improves children's language and communication skills, and aids their personal development. Sophie started going to Speech and Language Therapy in May 2011 when she was just 5 months old. Again they did not know much about microtia, so they were depending on Fiona to enlighten them! They took Sophie's history and did several tests with sounds using drums and maracas etc. Sophie's reactions were very good so they were well pleased with that. They also gave Fiona a leaflet with general advice on activities to encourage Sophie's communication development.

This brings me to the help that you as a parent can also provide for your child. Probably one of the most important sources of help for your child with microtia, is the help you can give them in their everyday activities. Do not leave it all to the professionals. They are vital and can help you a lot but you are the person that spends most time with your child. You are the one who has to ensure that your child wears their Baha properly throughout the day. You are the one that your child follows and copies. A child with normal hearing develops their speech and language through this naturally, but a child with microtia needs that extra help, time and effort from their parents. So what can you do? Sophie's therapist was a lady called Patrice Mahon. She gave Fiona some very useful pointers for helping Sophie at home. I will outline these briefly to give you an idea of the simple things that can be done.

1. Keep your language simple.
2. Draw attention to sounds and tell them what it is every time.

3. Talk about everything - I am washing your arms.

4. Speak slowly.

5. Always respond when your child makes a sound, by copying it.

6. Repeat words over and over e.g. 'bottle'

7. Use actions and gestures.

8. Sing nursery rhymes.

9. Look at books together.

10. Use familiar words often e.g. 'bye-bye', 'no', 'up' and 'Sophie'.

As parents, you are the most important people in your child's development and learning. The way you talk and play with them can make a big difference. Fiona was always very active in encouraging Sophie's development in the first 3 years and the proof of that is very clear to see in Sophie today.

Here in Lisburn, N Ireland, there is a Parent and Infant Project (PIP) run by Barnardo's, which is very helpful but I'm not sure about the availability of it in other parts of the UK. Referrals are usually accepted from Health Visitors, Social Workers, Speech Therapists and other professionals as well as self-referrals and referrals from community groups. The aims of this service are to enable young children to achieve their potential according to their abilities, to develop socially, emotionally, physically and intellectually and to establish an environment where parents will be facilitated in recognising and meeting the needs of their children. It aims to provide information to achieve a greater understanding of why children behave in certain ways. Parents have opportunities to learn about the importance of play, communication and language development. At PIP they use the High Scope model which is designed to enable young children to learn through direct experiences and provides opportunities to experiment and explore materials by themselves alongside a supportive adult. Children and adults work together as problem solvers, decision makers and planners.

Finally you need to know that in the UK there is financial support available too. Disability Living Allowance (DLA) for children under 16 years may help with the extra costs of looking after a child who needs more care than a child of the same age who does not have a disability. Many parents of children with microtia are receiving this. Of course your child will have to meet the eligibility requirements to qualify. Do look this up, it is worth a try!

There is another source of information that you might like to browse and that is Microtia Mingle UK on facebook. This is a closed group so you have to apply to join. Here you can meet and chat with other parents who also have children with microtia. It is a great place to meet people in similar situations and you will not feel so alone as you seek advice and discover things you might not have been aware of!

There is help out there so keep asking, and do use the Internet!

Chapter 6

Progress

We all thought that the two meetings in London would give us the information necessary to decide on the right route for Sophie. Well it did, but not in the way that we had hoped. So what was everyone's reaction to what was said at these two meetings? Fiona called me after seeing Dr Reinisch. She was cautiously upbeat. The main detail that caught my attention was that he had told them the drilling of the ear depended on the middle ear formation. Apparently it works on a scale of 1-10 and the level has to be at least 7 to justify an operation. If it falls below this, then it is really not effective. He said the scan of her ears would take place when she was around 2 years old. I admit that I did feel a bit concerned but still quietly confident that Sophie would be at the right end of the scale. Fiona and Colin really believe that Sophie can hear some things without the Baha, so our hope is that the middle ear is good. It was going to be a lot of money for all the treatment but I was convinced we would get the money from somewhere. This was positive!

Now I just had to wait and hear what Mr Bulstrode had to say. I really wanted it to be as positive as the first meeting because obviously London is closer to home. Again Fiona called me straight after the meeting and the main point that came from it was that they do not drill out an ear canal in GOSH, nor do they do it anywhere in the UK! He was amazed that they had thought it was going to happen. I was gutted to say the least, but I am still thinking everything is fine because we can go to the USA. Fiona said that Mr Bulstrode explained that with microtia the middle ear does not form properly and drilling will not improve the hearing! The operation he performs is for cosmetic ears only, made from cartilage at around 9-10 years old, and hearing aids will always be necessary! He also said there was no need for a scan as it is pointless. Fiona and Colin were in shock and I just could not get to grips with it. My stomach sank, how did we get it so wrong? Who led us to believe differently? Why was everything going wrong?

I had very mixed feelings and felt sad for Sophie. Then I asked myself why. She is a very happy little girl. She does not know any other way. This is normality for her. We are the ones that are not happy with the situation. Yes, we all only want what is best for her, but is pushing this little girl through all these operations in the USA what really is best for her? The doubt set in and a lot of thinking had to be done along with a lot more reading up on the Internet.

Finally Fiona and Colin realized that there were many problems associated with Dr Reinisch's methods. Not everyone came out with a new canal and new ears and able to hear as normal, without complications. It was time to give up on that dream and concentrate on getting Sophie the best hearing aids possible so that her hearing was the best it could be and her speech could develop normally. I was sceptical and I was worried if this was at all possible. Sophie was still only 8 months old and it was too early to know what she would be able to achieve, but we had to believe that it would all work out in the end. So where do we go from here......how do we help Sophie achieve the best hearing possible and set her up for a prosperous and happy future?

At this young age the important thing was to make sure Sophie could hear as well as could be expected, that she had continuous support from as many providers as possible and that she led a normal life.

In October 2011 Fionnuala McCreanor, Perapatetic Teacher of Hearing Impaired Children, provided her first support plan for Sophie. This service offered by SEELB (South Eastern Education and Library Board in Northern Ireland) has proved to be, and still is, such a valuable provision, continuing to play a crucial role in Sophie's development and well-being.

The initial plan outlined the provision of all her needs and targets as follows:

- Establish regular use of Baha
- Provide information to the parents
- Develop understanding of hearing levels, audiogram and audiology
- Develop understanding of foundations of language

- Establish hearing thresholds using free-field testing
- Discuss strategies towards development of first words

These targets were to be achieved through regular home visits, the checking and maintaining of equipment and continued liaison with ENT at the Royal Victoria Hospital and Speech and Language Therapy.

Understanding audiograms and hearing loss is quite difficult but try and keep the following in mind. The degree in hearing loss is expressed by the difference between a person's threshold and the average threshold for people of normal sensitivity. For example, persons with mild hearing loss have thresholds that are 25-30 dB higher than the thresholds for those with normal hearing when tested at several frequencies. Thresholds of 0-25 dB are quite normal for adults and 0-15 dB is normal for children.

For a brief moment I need to squeeze in some news! In early 2012, Fiona and Colin announced that Sophie was going to have a little brother or sister in November! This was great news and everyone was so excited for them. Of course they wondered if this baby would have microtia too, but the prospect did not frighten them at all. They said it would not be any different having one or two children with the same condition and at least they would be well prepared!

Sophie's first Progress Report from Fionnuala came in May 2012 when she was 17 months old. The audiology information provided stated that the results of the ABR* test showed a conductive hearing loss of 55-60 dB, while bone conduction thresholds were 10-20 dB.

*ABR test: The ABR test measures the reaction of the parts of a child's nervous system that affect hearing. It is a helpful tool in determining a child's ability to hear. The test uses a special computer to measure the way the child's hearing nerve responds to different sounds. Three to four small stickers called 'electrodes' are placed on the child's head and in front of his or her ears and connected to a computer. As sounds are made through the earphones, the electrodes measure how the child's hearing nerves respond to them. When Paediatric Warble Tone was used at home, Sophie responded consistently at approximately 20 db across the frequency range.

It was all good. Her developmental progress was within normal limits. At this stage Sophie was walking and her balance was good. She was interested in her environment and was responsive and alert to what she saw happening around her. She had good eye contact and was vocalising like a normal baby of this age. In general it was reported that Sophie's play skills were well developed, also she was very social and engaged readily with others in play. Early Monitoring Protocol monitors areas of development and her milestones appeared to be developing within normal limits. In May 2012 the following levels were noted:

Chronological age: 17 months

Communication, Attending and Listening, Social-Emotional and Play were equivalent to approximately 18 months. Vocalisation was 15-18 months.

This was a very positive report and the sense of support and not being alone was such a comfort to us all.

Meanwhile all went well with the birth of our fourth grandchild. The little boy arrived on 20th November 2012. He was a big baby weighing in at 9lbs 6.5ozs (4.27kg), and he did not have microtia! Sophie was delighted with her new brother Caleb and loved 'helping' mum in every way a 2 year old found possible!

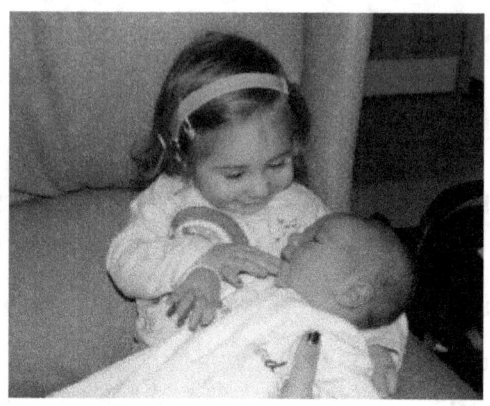

Figure 10: Sophie and Caleb

Christmas came and went and 2013 appeared. Sophie's speech was developing very well, and to be honest much better than I ever anticipated. This was such an important development in her journey with microtia. Sophie wore her hearing aid religiously every day. She was discharged from speech therapy which made her mum and dad very proud! Her progress was being monitored by regular reviews with their consultant Mr Trimble, who plans her way forward. The next big step will be having an implant for her hearing aid, which is usually done around the age of four when the skull should be thick enough.

Fionnuala continued to work on updating her support plans. With Sophie starting playgroup in

September, new targets and strategies were presented as follows in February 2013:

Targets:
- Monitor responses with new BAHA
- Establish listening levels using free-field testing
- Continue to develop early language skills: naming objects, looking at books
- Continue to develop speech and language skills: expressive, receptive language
- Continue to develop play skills, e.g. taking turns, imaginative play, matching
- Develop auditory processing skills

Strategies:
- Regular home visits
- Check and maintain equipment
- Liaison with ENT, RVH and Speech and Language Therapist
- Early Monitoring Protocol

The next progress report came in June 2013 at age 2 years 6 months. It stated that Sophie's receptive and expressive language was developing within normal limits. She was communicating easily with others and was able to express her own needs without always needing her parents help. It was noted that Sophie's speech was easy to understand, although she did appear to have a slight 'nasal' quality to some of her words. This was to be monitored with ENT. The following are the levels reported in May 2013 when using the Early Monitoring Protocol:

Chronological age: 2 years 5 months.

Communication, Attending and Listening, Vocalisation, Social-Emotional, other developmental milestones and play were all at a level of approximately 30 months. This was a very pleasing and satisfactory result!

At the end of September 2013 there was more good news for Sophie. She was offered the opportunity to trial bilateral hearing aids to see if they brought any improvement to her directional sound. It was hoped that there would be other advantages too like selective listening and better understanding in noisy situations. This was a very exciting development in the journey to improve Sophie's hearing! Over the next few months Fiona noticed a huge improvement in her hearing. She started to show some directional responses to sound and was now relying heavily on both hearing aids for that increase in quality. If one turns off or falls off she would say she could not hear properly!

It was always such a delight to hear how Sophie was progressing. This was a normal little girl who loved books, music, dancing and role play and microtia was appearing to be insignificant in her development. After being monitored frequently on communication, attending and listening, vocalisation and social-emotional skills, her developmental milestones were within normal limits.

In October 2013 Sophie started Busy Bees playgroup for two afternoons each week. Fionnuala continued her valued support by visiting her at playgroup and observing how she was settling in. The playgroup leader reported that initially she was quiet but slowly became more confident. This was a worrying time for her mum and dad as she was being thrown into a situation where there were lots of other children and an abundance of noise. It probably was a bit scary for her at first until she got used to it, but eventually she came out of her shell and seemed to be enjoying the experience! Fionnuala noted that Sophie was responding more confidently when wearing both Bahas. It enabled her to localise sound and her listening skills were very good during storytelling.

When deciding if a child with bilateral hearing impairment would benefit from wearing two hearing aids, I think the only way to find out is to give that child a chance to try it before a decision is made on implants. Two hearing aids have got to be better than one!

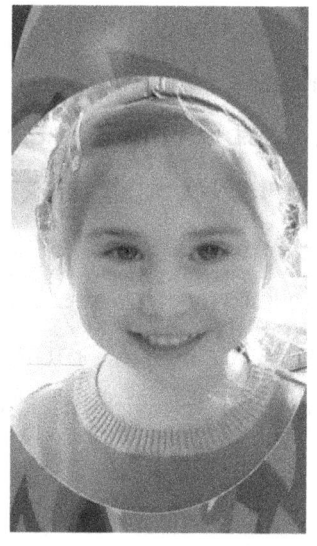

Figure 11: Happy girl with two Bahas!

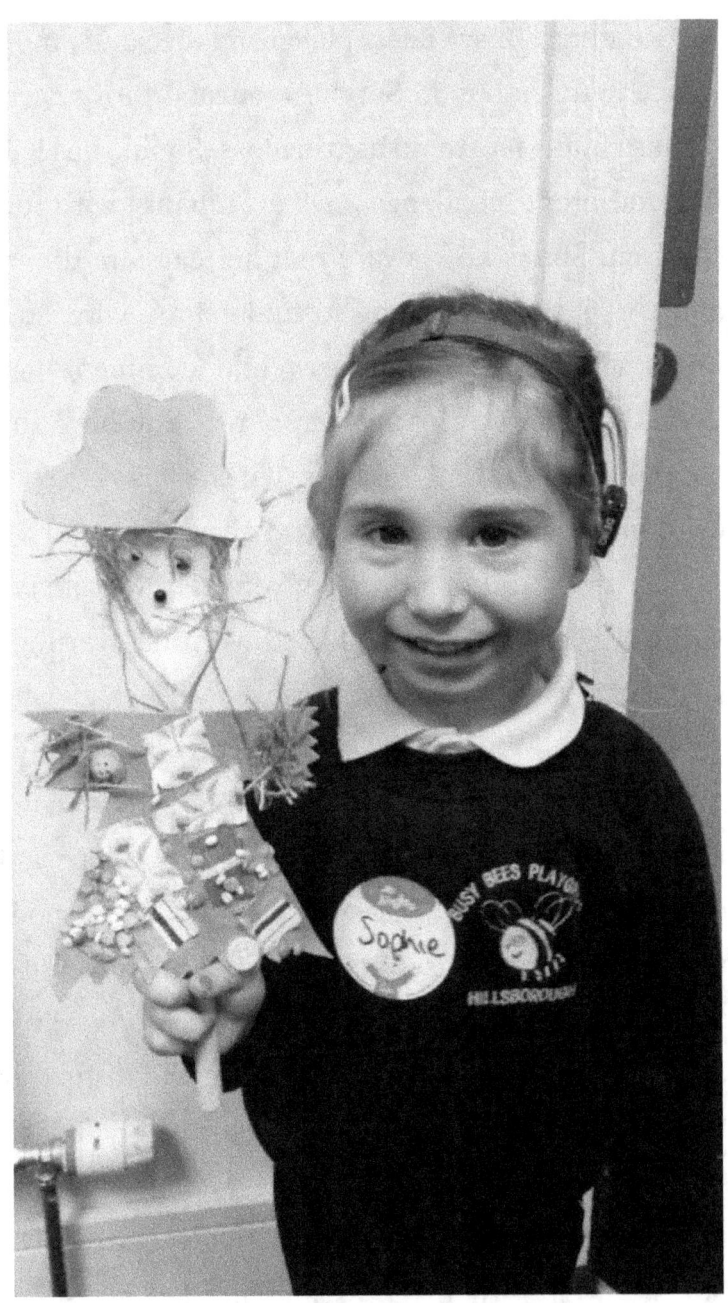

Figure 12: Having fun at playgroup

Attending Busy Bees playgroup became another welcome milestone in Sophie's journey with microtia. Unlike children with no hearing loss, Sophie has had to face different challenges when mixing with other children. She is now aware that her ears are different and she is still too young to understand why, so she finds it hard when another child comments with, "What is wrong with your ears?" or, "You have funny ears." We have always told her that she has very special ears and she appears willing to accept that for now. This brings to mind a little conversation we had when she and her brother once stayed with me overnight. I wear contact lenses as I have very bad short-sightedness. When I get up in the morning I wear glasses for a while and then change to my contact lenses. Sophie had never seen me do this before and of course was very inquisitive. I told her I could not see very well and the lenses helped me to see more clearly. She asked me why I was not able to see properly so I explained that lots of people are born with little things that are different and that they may need help with. I said that in the same way she could not hear well with her ears and needed hearing aids to hear better, I could not see well with my eyes and needed glasses and contact lenses to see better. I also explained that Granda could not walk very well because his legs were too weak so he needed a wheelchair to help him get around. Sophie thought all this was wonderful and the expression on her face told me that she understood completely and accepted that these things just happen.

I find this little grandchild of mine totally amazing! She is beautiful inside and out, she is funny and she is adorable. But I do get upset at times when I think of the challenges she will be facing throughout her life. When writing this book I promised to myself that I would be honest. This is one of those moments. This may sound wrong but there are times when I look at her ears and I have a moment of sadness and wish that she did not have microtia. It is that protectiveness coming out in a Granny who knows how harsh life can be and wants to shield her grandchildren from harm. Don't get me wrong, it is not that I think Sophie is imperfect, she is perfect to me and would not be any more perfect if she did not have microtia. I am very proud of her but I do worry about her.

March 2014 brought another quite different and strange issue to my daughter and her family, which fits in well with my story in the last couple of paragraphs!

Sophie's brother Caleb who was then 16 months old developed an infection in his eye which became a worry when it gradually spread to his cheek and ear. The GP was a bit concerned and sent him to the Royal Hospital. They confirmed it was an infection but decided to do a chest X-ray to make sure the infection had not spread. The X-ray showed the most amazing thing..... Caleb's heart was on the opposite side! At first they were not sure if it was just the heart but further scans showed that all of his organs were the 'opposite way round'. In fact his body was a mirror image of 'normality'! This was a total shock as none of us had ever heard of this! On further consultation and a lot of googling we discovered this was a rare condition called Situs Inversus Totalis found in only about 0.01% of the population. It involves complete transposition (right to left reversal) of all of the abdominal organs. However this is the most common form of the condition in that it usually causes no medical problems and life goes on as normal. Apparently it can be an issue if only the heart or some of the organs are reversed. So after the initial shock of hearing this, we were all able to relax and accept it was not going to cause Caleb any problems. They did say they would see him in a year for a check-up and having had this done in 2015, the consultant was very happy and did not wish to see him again. So after my little conversation with Sophie we were able to add Caleb to the group of people who are born with little things that are different!

Sophie finished her playgroup year in June 2014. Fionnuala carried out a Progress Report in January of that year. When assessed at home Sophie can respond at 30/40 dB across the frequency range. Fionnuala uses the McCormick Toy Test* to determine the quality and levels of hearing impairment. It consists of 14 paired words and is ideal for children with a mental age of 2 years plus.

*The test was developed by Professor Barry McCormick OBE (Director – retired, Children's Hearing and Assessment Centre, Nottingham) and was first published in 1977. It is widely used in clinics and hospitals as an effective way of identifying hearing difficulties in young children aged 18 months plus.

The McCormick Toy discrimination test uses 14 paired words, which are generally recognized by children from an early age. Each word in the list has a matching item in the set and a paired item with a similar vowel or diphthong, but differing consonants.

TREE	KEY
SHOE	SPOON
COW	HOUSE
PLANE	PLATE
HORSE	FORK
DUCK	CUP
MAN	LAMB

The child is asked to identify each toy, and any not identified are removed from the test. The child is placed in front of the toys and asked, "show me the ...." This is requested at differing sound levels and a child with normal hearing should be able to discriminate between items at a listening level of 40 dBA. The criteria for passing this test is when a child gives four correct responses out of five requests. Current recommendations are that any child who cannot pass the test at 40 dBA should be referred to a specialist Audiology Centre. (The 'A' means adjusted levels).

The advantage of this test is that it is very simple. Parents and teachers can immediately see the natural confusion which can arise when a child has a slight hearing difficulty. Sophie was able to firstly name 13 out of 14 items. Initially she did not know 'lamb' but when told it she repeated it and could remember what it was. At 60 dBA and with no lip reading Sophie scored 14/14. At 45 dBA and with no lip reading she scored 11/14. These scores would indicate a pass and suggest that Sophie's hearing, with both Bahas, is within acceptable limits.

At playgroup it was found that Sophie was progressing well and the staff reported no concerns. Sophie effectively uses language to explore and understand her world; for instance she will ask questions and will talk alone during play. Her speech is easy to understand but she still has a slight nasal quality to some of her words. It has been noted that Sophie does not always pronounce the letter 's', however when her attention is drawn to it she can generally correct it. When seen at RVH it was found that her adenoids were fine so were not responsible for her leaving out the letter 's'. It appears then that it is a 'learned behaviour' and hopefully with encouragement she can correct it.

Early Monitoring Protocol was used to monitor areas of development. Sophie's play skills and developmental milestones appeared to be within normal limits. In November 2013 when she was 2 years 11 months old all her developmental milestones were equivalent to 36 months.

For me the value and continuity of the work carried out by Fionnuala and the Service for the Sensory Impaired cannot be underestimated. It puts all of us more at ease when we know we can rely on their support and work.

Sophie is now approaching the age for implants and if you are not familiar with what they are I will use this opportunity to explain.

Cochlear™ provide two implant systems, the Baha® Attract and the Baha® Connect, which do away with the need for a headband. In both systems the implant is the same, in the form of a small screw which is implanted into the bone. The Baha Attract uses an internal and external magnet to connect the sound processor to the implant. The invisible connection is discreet and appealing and sets a new standard in the hearing experience. The Baha Connect snaps on to an abutment which is fixed on to the implant. There are two types of abutment: one is Titanium, the other has a Hydroxyapitite coating and is the one that Fiona and Colin chose for Sophie. It is a matter of personal choice when it comes to deciding which system you think would be best for your child. More information on these systems can be found on the Cochlear website.

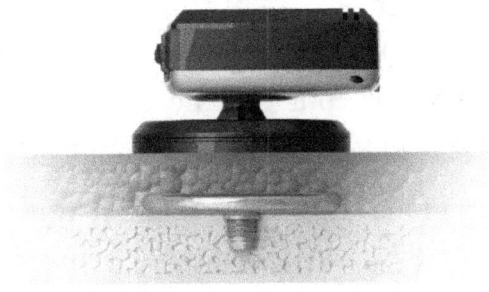

Figure 13: BAHA Attract (image courtesy of Cochlear™)

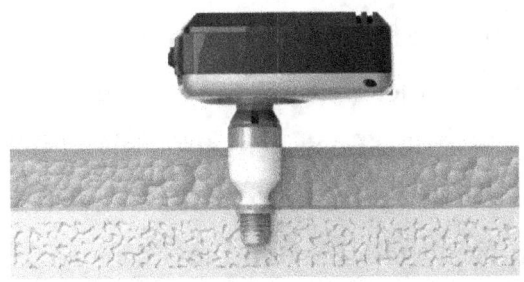

Figure 14: BAHA Connect (image courtesy of Cochlear™)

Meeting with the consultant gave Fiona and Colin a lot to think about. Bilateral microtia is rarer then unilateral microtia and Mr Trimble has only ever implanted on one side. This is what he knows best and wants to do with Sophie. Bilateral implants have never before been carried out in Northern Ireland. But my daughter has different ideas because she observes daily how Sophie relies on both of her present hearing aids, and she has seen the improvements that two Bahas have made. Fiona knew it could be done and felt very strongly about it, but she needed to convince Mr Trimble! The operation can be done in one or two stages but Fiona and Colin wanted him to implant bilaterally and in one operation!

Fiona decided to discuss it with Fionnuala and get her opinion as she has been following Sophie all the way. She was totally in agreement and in May 2014 she sent a letter to Mr Trimble outlining the benefits of two Bahas for Sophie. Her initial concern was that Sophie would be starting Busy Bees Pre-School in September and it would be a very busy environment with approximately 26 other children there. In this situation she believed it would be difficult for Sophie to hear and understand her teacher, particularly during group activities. Localising sound would be a big problem with one Baha. Furthermore when Sophie starts her formal education in Primary School she reckoned it would be harder for her to pick out speech sounds from competing background noise and she could miss information or instructions being given out in class. Fionnuala quite rightly pointed out that schools are a much different environment than in the past, in that the majority of learning happens through group work where a lot of discussion and conversation is taking place. She feared that because Sophie was already a very able and bright child, she could become anxious if unable to follow what was happening around her. This in turn could adversely affect her academic progress.

Sophie's parents only want what is best for her. There are many decisions to be made for her as she is too young to make them herself. The best start possible in her educational pathway was their main priority at this stage and that depended on their decision. They still had doubts. Maybe the consultant was right; should Sophie just have one implant fitted now and wait for further developments in technology? There are so many questions without answers. But in the end Fionnuala's support for implanting the two Bahas gave them the confidence that they were doing the right thing and I totally backed them on this.

So it was back to Mr Trimble with their thoughts and feelings and next thing they knew they were signing the papers. Sophie was now on the waiting list for bilateral implants and she would be the first child in Northern Ireland to have this type of operation! Sophie was very excited at the thought of not having to wear a headband anymore. Her mum told her she was having 'diamonds' put into her bone (because it sounded much more appealing than screws!) and she would be able to click her hearing aids on to them.

September 3rd 2014, the big day arrived and Sophie was brilliant! She was very brave and sailed through the operation with no problems. Everything went smoothly but the skull was a bit thinner than expected.

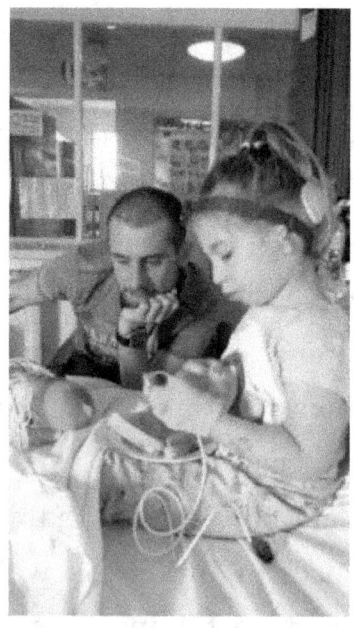

Figure 15: Sophie after bilateral implant surgery

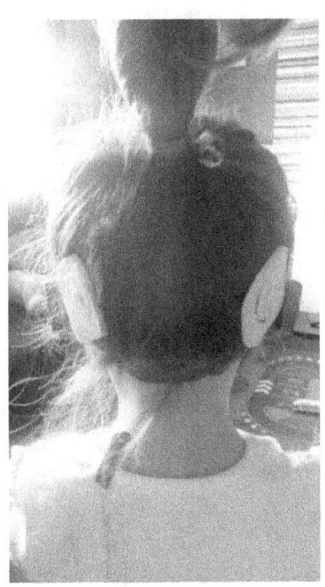

Figure 16: Sophie showing off her new implants

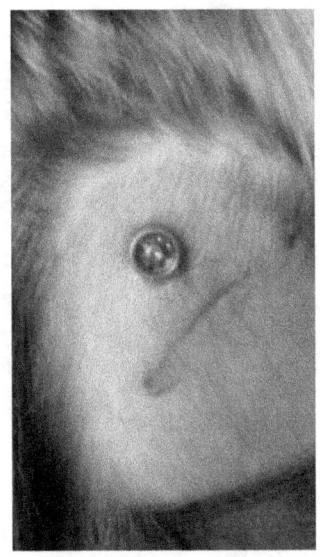

Figure 17: Close-up of abutment

Mr Trimble advised them that they would have to wait longer than usual to have the sound processor connected up. In the meantime Sophie had to continue wearing her headband to allow time for the healing process. She started her Busy Bees Pre-school year and settled well while waiting to 'go live' with her hearing aid connection which was proposed for the end of November.

October 4th 2014 brought a big adventure for me. I set off for Australia for 4 weeks to visit my second eldest daughter Melanie, husband Sam and little Sienna who was just 10 weeks old, and my only son Simon who lives out there too. Unfortunately I went alone as my husband was unable to travel due to his MS. It was difficult leaving the rest of my family (I have two daughters and four grandchildren here), but Melanie had had a rough time with Sienna's birth and it was time to focus on her family for a while and give them some support too! As far as I was concerned Sophie had come a long way and was doing well and hopefully by the time I got back the headband would have disappeared for good!

It was mid-October and we were in a beautiful place called Byron Bay on the East coast of Australia. We went there for 9 days to spend some time with Simon who was in the process of opening up a Toastie Bar! While we were there Fiona sent me a text to let me know that one of Sophie's screws had fallen out. She was devastated. I managed to call her by phone and she said that Sophie just woke up and found it on the pillow. This was a big blow and there was now a concern that the other one might come out as well. At this stage she was trying to get an urgent meeting with the consultant so there was nothing else to do but wait and see. There was no disguising the disappointment in her voice and unfortunately there was nothing I could say or do to ease this. There was also the guilt of wondering should they have pushed for the bilateral operation or stuck with Mr Trimble's first plan, but I assured her this could have happened even if there had been just one implant.

When they met Mr Trimble he said that it probably came out because the bone was a bit too thin and his only hope was that the other one would remain intact. He said there was nothing could be done and the bone would have to be left to heal and hopefully strengthen, then he would try the implant again at a later stage. My concern on hearing this news was that he had operated too soon at 3 years 9 months old. Maybe another 6 months would have made a difference but who knows.

So Sophie after all ends up with one implant and not the two that they fought for and felt was necessary for her quality of hearing. This was going to be a challenge for her. She was so happy to be getting rid of the headband so how would she feel if she had to wear it again for the second hearing aid....

Chapter 7

Moving On

No matter what life throws at us we all have to move on to the best of our capability and that is exactly what had to be done when things did not go according to plan after Sophie's operation.

Sophie had to wear her headband for the first couple of months at Busy Bees nursery. She was eventually 'linked up' on 7th December 2014 and was delighted she had at last got rid of the headband. A few technical adjustments were made and she was ready to go! Her hearing appeared to be really good, which was expected because the sound pathway is now directly into the bone rather than through the flesh barrier. When probed about needing the second hearing aid Sophie insisted that she could hear well enough without it! So that was that and she seemed to manage well enough throughout her nursery year with no problems.

Fionnuala continued to monitor her by visiting her in the classroom and observing how she was coping with everything. She changed her support plan as Sophie progressed. In February 2015 her targets and strategies were set as follows:

- Monitor responses with one Baha. Observation of localisation skills
- Establish listening levels using free-field testing
- Continue to monitor language skills and develop auditory processing skills
- Regular home visits
- Regular visits to nursery
- Check and maintain equipment
- Liaison with ENT, RVH and Speech and Language Therapist
- Assessments: BPVS*

*BPVS is the British Picture Vocabulary Scale used for children 3 to 16 years. It is a test of receptive (hearing) vocabulary, i.e. single words that a child can understand. The questions broadly sample words that represent a range of content areas such as actions, animals, toys and emotions and parts of speech such as nouns, verbs or attributes, across all levels of difficulty. Basically, the tester says a word and the child responds by selecting the picture (from four options) that best illustrates the word's meaning. The test gives a standard score, percentile rank and age equivalent for the child's level of receptive vocabulary. This means that the child's score can be compared with that of hearing children of the same age. In September 2014, Sophie's speech and language was assessed using the British Picture Vocabulary Scale and the result was as follows:

Chronological Age: 3 years 9 months

Age Equivalent: 3 years 3 months

Sophie got through her nursery year very well and Fionnuala's progress report in June 2015 reflected that, although we must remember that it is not all plain sailing! Since being fitted with the external part of her Baha in December, early responses have been encouraging. She is noticing sounds that she was unable to pick up before, for example a car driving past their home. Sophie says she loves her new hearing aid and proudly shows it off! As I said before she prefers to wear her new Baha only, but the option of the second Baha on the softband is there should she change her mind.

However, using performance testing, Fionnuala says it is evident Sophie is listening from one side only and she turns to her implanted side at all times, even if a sound or voice is presented on her non-implanted side. Fiona has noted that when assessed at ENT she responded in the same manner. Fionnuala believes this would be a concern for localisation when she starts Primary School in September.

The McCormick Toy Test was carried out again and Sophie was able to name 14/14 items (aided). At 60 dBA and with no lip reading Sophie scored 14/14, and at 45 dBA with no lip reading she scored 11/14. This indicated a pass, as in the previous test, and suggested that Sophie's hearing, with her implanted Baha, is within acceptable limits at this time. Fionnuala is still concerned that Sophie will have difficulty with localisation in the classroom, particularly with 30 children.

Regarding communication, at this stage Sophie's receptive and expressive language appeared to be developing within normal limits. She was able to communicate easily with others and could express her own needs independently. She had a keen interest in things happening around her and could absorb new ideas. She could retell past events and stories and react appropriately to complex questions. Although her speech continued to be easy to understand, she was not always pronouncing the letters 's' and 'f' correctly, but when this was pointed out to her, with encouragement she was able to rectify this. At this stage the slight nasal sound in her speech has now disappeared!

Fionnuala concluded that Sophie's developmental progress appears to be within normal limits. She remains an alert child, has good eye contact and vocalises readily. She is confident and has great empathy to others and an awareness of how her actions may impact others. Sophie has a passion for books and she is excellent at jigsaw puzzles. Her imaginary play skills show lots of detail and she also enjoys active play.

I am very impressed with the support Sophie continues to get from Fionnuala and the Service for the

Sensory Impaired. It is so valuable for Sophie's development and it makes me feel very content that someone out there really cares so much about hearing impaired children in such a structured and passionate way. I see a little girl developing normally with only minor issues arising as a result of her microtia. She continues to amaze me and rarely complains about or questions her condition. I do not think we can ever complain about the lack of support she has had, and continues to have, from all sources.

So all is going well but there is still the issue of the second abutment coming out. At the time Fiona wanted it redone straightaway and Colin thought it was better to wait. I can understand Fiona's concern and frustration but I also thought it was better to wait for a while especially if it fell out because the bone was too thin. In the end they decided to think about it again after Christmas. In early 2015 they went to see Mr Trimble who decided to put Sophie on the waiting list for surgery. He said there was a long waiting time so he would put her down as urgent. The idea was that she would have the surgery done and the link-up complete and settled before she started school in September. Fiona believed that having two hearing aids would give

Sophie the best start possible and provide her with much better directional sound, which seemed to be an issue at times.

Time went on and finally in April 2015 Sophie had to go for a pre-op assessment. Mr Trimble assured them Sophie was still on the urgent waiting list and it should not be too long until she was called. Fiona badly wanted this operation well before Sophie started school but it did not happen. She finally got the appointment for the surgery to take place at the beginning of September, just when she was due to start school! It was a long, long wait and unfortunately the operation was going to disrupt her first and very important days at school. This caused a lot of stress for her parents as they wanted the best possible start for Sophie. She attended her new school Meadowbridge Primary for one week initially, had the operation and was off school for a full week. Everything seemed to go well and Sophie settled into school again, much easier than we expected. (We do worry unnecessarily sometimes!)

There are many big decisions to be taken when you have a child with specific needs, and these decisions have to be made with the best interests of the child at heart. You only get 'one go' at it and you want to get it right first time. Sophie was going into her new school with only one Baha so Fiona and Colin had to be sure she was able to hear at the best possible level from Day One. As Fionnuala provides Sophie's educational support, she had no doubt whatsoever that Sophie would now benefit from a Digital Hearing Aid system (provided by the Education Board and not the NHS), to allow her to hear her teacher more easily above the classroom noise. For all children, especially those with hearing difficulties, it's important to hear well at school. Classrooms are a dynamic place for interaction and of course learning. In order to fully participate, every child needs to hear not only the teacher, but also classmates and multimedia devices within the classroom. The 'Roger for Education' accessories provide a solution for every situation. Sometimes hearing through a hearing aid in general is not helpful enough if the sound you are listening to continues to relocate or move away from you. For example, when a teacher is speaking in front of a child who wears a hearing aid, that child can hear great, until the teacher moves away from that child and walks to the other side of the classroom. When a teacher wears an FM system microphone (connecting with the receiver end on the child's hearing aid), the child can then hear just fine no matter where the teacher moves about the classroom. As the teacher speaks into the microphone her voice is transmitted directly into the child's ear or bone through their hearing aid. It is as if the teacher is always standing directly in front of the child while teaching at any spot in the classroom.

For Sophie a 'Phonak' Dynamic Radio System with a Roger transmitter and receiver is used.

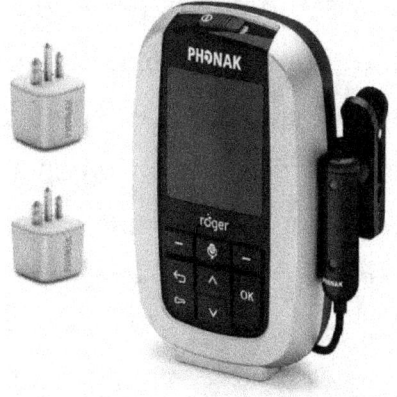

Figure 18: Phonak radio system

The transmitter is like a mobile phone and the microphone is attached to it by a lead. If the teacher wears the transmitter round the neck, the microphone can be clipped to the neck cord. Some teachers prefer to clip the transmitter to their belt and then clip the microphone to their tie, shirt or other clothing. The receiver is then plugged into Sophie's Baha processor. This receiver is very small measuring 9 x 9 x 12 mm and weighing 1.205 g! My daughter tells me that Sophie and her teacher call the transmitter and receiver Roger and Regina! Sophie is very independent and takes charge of the plugging in and removal of the receiver during each school day. It is kept in a box behind the teacher's desk and every morning Sophie goes and gets it. She removes her Baha and plugs in the receiver and at the end of the day she removes it and puts it back in the box! What a responsibility for a little 5 year old girl to have, and she manages it so well and wants to do it herself! There was an occasion when she forgot to put it back and Fiona noticed it while travelling home from school in the car. Now Fiona checks her every day when she comes out of school to make sure she has removed it and if she has forgotten to remove it she gives it to the teacher. Fiona says she likes to make sure it is safely in the classroom as it is very expensive and she does not want to be responsible for losing it!

Another support plan came from Fionnuala in October 2015 just after Sophie started school at 4 years 9 months. The same targets and strategies to monitor Sophie were in place as in the previous plan, including the BPVS assessment.

I am delighted that Sophie has been given the best start in Primary School, especially when she was depending on only one Baha for hearing. But with the 'switch-on' of the second Baha being due on 7th December 2015 there came more bad news. The implant did not 'take' again. It eventually became loose and fell out in October. This was devastating news for all of us and it was an even bigger blow when her parents were told that she would have to wait for a couple of years before they would think of implanting again. So unfortunately Sophie has not been able to experience the advantages of having two implant systems, even though she was the first person in Northern Ireland to have the bilateral operation. There has been a lot of worry, disappointment and despair over this setback, but in the end you have to move on and play with the hand you have been dealt. As I said before, we are the worriers, not Sophie. This very happy little granddaughter of mine just takes it all in her stride and is dealing with it amazingly!

In April 2016 when Sophie was 5 years 4 months old Fionnuala's report conveyed some very encouraging test results that stood out for us:

<u>British Picture Vocabulary Scale</u>: age equivalent 6 years

<u>Renfrew Action Picture Test</u>: age equivalent for Grammar 6 years to 6 years 6 months, and for Information 7 years to 7 years 6 months

<u>Renfrew Vocabulary Test</u>: age equivalent 5 years to 5 years 6 months

What more could we ask for!

Chapter 8

Looking Ahead

Sophie is now 5 years 6 months old and she has almost finished her first year in Primary School. Her progress reports from Fionnuala continue to be very encouraging. Sophie's hearing was assessed in this year in primary school and the responses for bone conduction indicated that her hearing levels were within normal limits. Results from ENT showed similar responses. In tests for Discrimination of Speech using the McCormick Toy Test (with the left Baha) her scores were as follows:

At 60 dBA and with no lip reading Sophie scored 14/14. At 45 dBA and with no lip reading Sophie scored 14/14. These scores indicate a pass and suggest that Sophie's hearing, with her implanted Baha, is within acceptable limits at this time.

Regarding receptive and expressive language she can communicate easily with others and is easily understood. She is quite capable of retelling simple past events, using age-appropriate language, and can answer questions giving full and detailed answers. Occasionally Sophie still does not pronounce the letters 's' and 'f' properly. However when her attention is drawn to this, she can generally correct it. For instance, when naming a 'shop', initially Sophie said 'hop'. However when her contribution was repeated back to her she laughed and self-corrected immediately saying, "No! I mean the shop!" Fionnuala feels, as Fiona does, that this may be a learned behaviour and with encouragement Sophie should, over time, continue to self-correct this. As Fionnuala has monitored her throughout the school year, she feels she has clearly benefitted from a structured environment and excellent teaching which ensures her educational needs are being met. Sophie's hearing levels are constantly monitored and reviewed and any concerns are reported immediately by her class teacher. The Digital Radio system is used when necessary by the teacher and also in assembly, and Sophie can alert someone if it is not operating properly. The staff at the school have received training in hearing impairment and are aware of the educational implications of her moderate, conductive hearing loss.

We have an assurance by Fionnuala that Sophie will continue to be supported by the Service for the Sensory Impaired and the degree of support given will be based on a recognised Criteria of Support. She will continue to be monitored in school and the staff will be kept updated on her hearing needs.

In this book I have covered more than 5 years of Sophie's life with microtia. I have also tried to include as much as possible on this condition, and the areas surrounding it. My daughter has picked up a lot of information along the way that she never would have known about, so I have tried to offer you, as readers, as much help as I possibly can, by telling Sophie's story from all angles and incorporating everything we as a family have learned over the years.

As I said before, you as parents will have to make

some tough decisions for your child as they will not be capable while they are young. But there will come a time when they will have to make a big decision themselves about ear reconstruction. I believe that with the right support and information, this should be their decision in the end. I would not like to think that Sophie or any other child would be pressured into having 'new' ears just because their parents want them to have 'normal ears'. For me this would be wrong. I think the child should be given all the information and options available and it is then up to them to make the decision. And they will change their minds from time to time depending on the situation. Fiona asked Sophie recently if she would like new ears like hers. She got a bit upset and said she did not want new ears, she just wanted to keep her own. Fiona of course said this was fine. Then a few weeks later she approached Fiona with a pencil and asked if she could help her to tuck the pencil behind her ear. Fiona tried but unfortunately the pencil would not stay in place. She explained to Sophie that her ears were a bit too small. Then Sophie looked at her for a moment and said, "I think I will get new ears!"

So what have we learned? For me I think the main

thing is that children with microtia can live perfectly normal lives if they get the love and support they need from their family, in conjunction with all the support available outside of the family. It is not enough to simply accept that your child has microtia and hope that everything falls into place. You must push for all the help you can get to meet the needs of your child, so that they can be happy. You will then be happy that you did everything you could to make their lives as normal as possible.

Postscript

My intentions were that this book would be completed and ready for print during 2016. Unfortunately, however, things didn't work out that way. Everything had to be put on hold for a while when I developed a mysterious illness that took months to recover from. Along with that my husband had a couple of spells in hospital and my mum passed away. But something good did happen! Fiona and Colin had another little baby boy named Luca on 14th Dec 2015. So now Sophie has two crazy but lovable brothers to contend with!

Thankfully we are all 'up and running' again and I would like to finish off by giving you a little update on Sophie's last 2 years. Sophie has not yet been given another chance to get the second implant redone. She has had a CT scan which shows that some areas of the skull are a lot thinner than others and this is of major concern to the surgeon. The problem is where to place the abutment. It obviously cannot be implanted in the same area as before, so it looks like it will have to go either above or below the original site and where the bone is thick enough. For Fiona this creates a problem of not being in line with the current one. In the grand scale of things this may seem a trivial matter but I do understand Fiona's reasoning on it. However if there is an area which is not symmetrical to the other abutment, and the surgeon feels the bone is able to take it, then I think it's the only answer. The main goal is for Sophie to have a Baha on either side so that she has better directional hearing. This makes sense as we have two ears for a reason!

So this is the stage we are at in February 2018. There are still ups and downs but no matter what happens Sophie is growing up and getting on with life. She is doing well at school in all subjects and has a great passion for art and craft. Her teacher says she loves a challenge in her work. Sophie is thriving like any other child and has no problems with her hearing!

I will always remember just after Sophie was born and the traumatic appointment with the first ENT specialist. Fiona was very upset and emotional and Colin and I were trying to console her. I remember Colin's words so well. He said, "She <u>will</u> hear us Fiona." And he was right. Even with one Baha.

Acknowledgements

I would like to express my gratitude to the many people who saw me through this book; to all those who provided support, talked things over, read, wrote, offered advice, allowed me to quote their remarks and assisted in the editing, proofreading and design. A special thank you to Fiona and Colin for allowing me to share Sophie's story with the outside world. I hope by doing so it will help families that are living with microtia, and provide them with answers to questions similar to those that Fiona and Colin had when Sophie was born.

In addition I would like to acknowledge the following people and services for their permission to let me use valuable copyright material from books, websites, files, reports etc.

- FOI Team at Great Ormond Street Hospital for 'Microtia Information' adapted from an original leaflet produced by GOSH (July 2014).

- Fionnuala McCreanor from 'Service for the Hearing Impaired' for access to all Sophie's reports and progress.
- Dr Reinisch from the 'Cedars-Sinai Center for International Health' in Los Angeles for information and use of transcript of meeting with Fiona & Colin.
- Mr. Neil Bulstrode, Consultant Plastic and Reconstructive Surgeon at GOSH for information and use of transcript of meeting with Fiona & Colin.
- Maisie Milward for the stage 1 photos of her new ear, carried out by Mr Bulstrode.
- Cochlear® for information and photos. www.cochlear.com
- Phonak UK for information and photos. www.phonak.co.uk
- Children's Craniofacial Association, Dallas for 'A Guide to Understanding Microtia'. www.ccakids.com

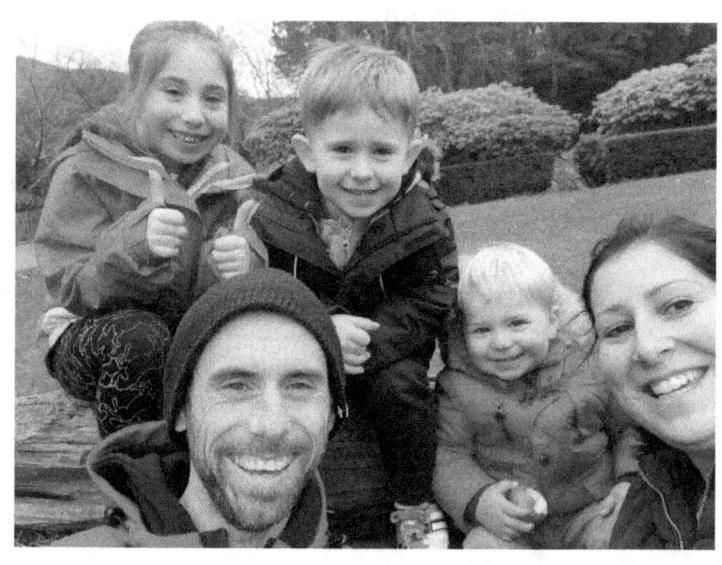

Fiona and Colin with Sophie, Caleb & Luca.

www.ingramcontent.com/pod-product-compliance
Lightning Source LLC
Chambersburg PA
CBHW071209240526
45470CB00018B/1649